first do no harm

BEING A RESILIENT DOCTOR
IN THE 21ST CENTURY

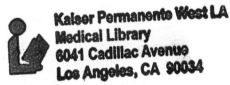

The McGraw·Hill Companies

First published 2009
Reprinted 2010 (twice)
Text © 2009 Acacia Arch Pty Ltd and Michael Kidd Pty Ltd
Illustrations and design © 2009 McGraw-Hill Australia Pty Ltd

National Library of Australia Cataloguing-in-Publication entry

Author:	Rowe, Leanne.
Title:	First do no harm: being a resilient doctor in the 21st century/ Leanne Rowe, Michael Kidd.
Edition:	1st ed.
ISBN:	9780070276970 (pbk.)
	9780070285583 (Special sale only)
Notes:	Includes index.
	Bibliography.
Subjects:	Physicians—Health and hygiene.
	Physicians—Mental health.
	Resilience (Personality trait).
	Self care, Health.
Other Authors/Contributors:	Kidd, Michael.
Dewey Number:	610.69

Published in Australia by
McGraw-Hill Australia Pty Ltd
Level 2, 82 Waterloo Road, North Ryde NSW 2113
Publisher: Elizabeth Walton
Managing Editor: Kathryn Fairfax
Production Editor: Emma Mullenger
Editor: Jennifer Coombs
Editorial Coordinator: Fiona Richardson
Proofreader: Terence Townsend
Indexer: Mary Coe, Potomac Indexing
Art Director: Astred Hicks
Internal design: Patricia McCallum
Cover design: Astred Hicks
Typeset in Australia by Midland Typesetters
Printed in China on 104 gsm woodfree recycled by iBook Printing Ltd

first do no harm

{first do no harm}

BEING A RESILIENT DOCTOR IN
THE 21ST CENTURY

LEANNE ROWE and MICHAEL KIDD

The **McGraw·Hill** Companies

Sydney New York San Francisco Auckland
Bangkok Bogotá Caracas Hong Kong
Kuala Lumpur Lisbon London Madrid
Mexico City Milan New Delhi San Juan
Seoul Singapore Taipei Toronto

The most essential resources doctors of all walks of the specialties bring with them are their interpersonal skills—the ability to relate to and care about the patient. That makes mental, emotional and physical fitness part of our competence profile. But medical practice can make for a stressful life, and most doctors tend to dodge, rather than confront this impact. This book provides leadership—in asking the right questions at the critical moment—or rather it promotes self-leadership in helping doctors to address a critical reflection of their fitness. 'First do no harm' starts with the preliminary 'do no harm to your own health as a doctor'. The interactive approach of this book is highly original and practical, in the quest for safer health care.

Professor Chris van Weel, President,
World Organization of Family Doctors (Wonca)

First do no harm goes beyond doctors' health and wellbeing. This inspiring book calls for a more supportive medical culture to assist us to become more resilient doctors. The issues raised are equally relevant for doctors across the globe.

Dr. Gabrielle Casper, immediate past
President of the Medical Women's International Association

About once a year, a doctor comes to me in distress: burnt out, disillusioned, embittered, full of self-doubt and perhaps suicidal. The worst thing about these doctors is that medicine, in whole or in part, in some way or other, usually lies at the root of the problem. The adage 'first, do no harm'—the need to reduce to zero the proportion of medical graduates who subsequently come to wish they had never owned a stethoscope—should be carved on the door of every medical admissions tutor, undergraduate teacher and postgraduate mentor. All would gain from reading this timely and thoughtful book from two of the acknowledged intellectual leaders of the profession.

Professor Trisha Greenhalgh OBE,
Professor of Primary Health Care, University College London

The perfect personal prescription for the busy doctor. The authors have simplified our complex daily lives and provided us with a toolkit for a health professional future.

Professor Deborah C Saltman AM, Institute of Postgraduate Medicine,
Brighton and Sussex Medical School, United Kingdom.

This is a wonderful resource that will make a real difference to the health and the effectiveness of medical practitioners. Finding balance and building resilience are the challenges for us all in our busy lives and this is just what the doctor ordered!

Dr Chris Mitchell, President,
Royal Australian College of General Practitioners

This book is essential reading for all doctors, especially those starting out. We need to be able to care for ourselves in order to be able to care for others effectively. This is a practical 'how to' guide and we should all be picking it up from time to time for a 'self-health' check.

Dr Desiree Yap, President, Australian Federation of Medical Women

Professional sustainability and wellbeing are ideas that resonate with the current generation of medical students and junior doctors. However they are lessons that are rarely learnt until later in our practicing lives.

Dr. Michael Bonning, past President of the Australian Medical Students Association and current member of the Australian Medical Association's Doctors in Training Committee

First, do no harm: being a resilient doctor in the 21st century *is an energising read at a time when the life of a doctor is increasingly demanding and stressful. Professor Leanne Rowe and Professor Michael Kidd have shown us the what, why and how of being a healthy and happy doctor to sustain our professional legacy. This book is a must-read for all doctors and medical students.*

Professor Cindy L.K. Lam, Head of Family Medicine,
The University of Hong Kong

I welcome this book as essential reading for all health professionals who wish to look after their own health and wellbeing, while taking care of others. This book complements the approach beyondblue *is taking in helping to strengthen practitioners' own resilience and mental health in their work environment. I commend the authors on this very important work.*

The Hon. Jeff Kennett, Chairman of *beyondblue*:
the national depression initiative (Australia)

This book is printed on recycled paper

DECLARATION OF GENEVA

AT THE TIME OF BEING ADMITTED AS A MEMBER OF THE MEDICAL PROFESSION:

I SOLEMNLY PLEDGE to consecrate my life to the service of humanity;

I WILL GIVE to my teachers the respect and gratitude that is their due;

I WILL PRACTISE my profession with conscience and dignity;

THE HEALTH OF MY PATIENT will be my first consideration;

I WILL RESPECT the secrets that are confided in me, even after the patient has died;

I WILL MAINTAIN by all the means in my power, the honour and the noble traditions of the medical profession;

MY COLLEAGUES will be my sisters and brothers;

I WILL NOT PERMIT considerations of age, disease or disability, creed, ethnic origin, gender, nationality, political affiliation, race, sexual orientation, social standing or any other factor to intervene between my duty and my patient;

I WILL MAINTAIN the utmost respect for human life;

I WILL NOT USE my medical knowledge to violate human rights and civil liberties, even under threat;

I MAKE THESE PROMISES solemnly, freely and upon my honour.

This declaration was written in response to medical crimes committed in World War II and declares our dedication to the humanitarian goals of medicine. It is a pledge to the higher calling of medicine and to human rights. Among these noble principles is the commitment to care for our colleagues as we care for our families.

Adopted by the 2nd General Assembly of the World Medical Association, Geneva, Switzerland, September 1948
and amended by the 22nd World Medical Assembly, Sydney, Australia, August 1968
and the 35th World Medical Assembly, Venice, Italy, October 1983
and the 46th WMA General Assembly, Stockholm, Sweden, September 1994
and editorially revised at the 170th Council Session, Divonne-les-Bains, France, May 2005 and the 173rd Council Session, Divonne-les-Bains, France, May 2006.

To our wonderful partners Peter Jasek and Alastair McEwin

ACKNOWLEDGMENTS

This book was developed with the support of many colleagues and friends. We greatly appreciate the support of Professor John Murtagh AM, our mentor, teacher and friend, who wrote the foreword to this book. We wish to acknowledge the following people who gave us constructive and valuable feedback through the writing process:

Professor Gavin Andrews AO, Dr Jill Benson, Dr Grant Blashki, Dr Michael Bonning, Dr Jan Coles, Dr Mukesh Haikerwal, Ms Beth Hewitt, Mr Chris Jasek, Dr Peter Jasek, Dr Jennifer Lonergan, Dr Ronald McCoy, Mr Alastair McEwin, Professor Helen Milroy, Associate Professor Marilyn McMurchie OAM, Professor Keryn Phelps, Professor Deborah Saltman AM, Associate Professor Peter Schattner, Ms Rosa Schattner, Ms Clare Shann, Dr Jill Tomlinson, Dr Beres Wenck, Dr Desiree Yap.

We also wish to thank all staff at McGraw-Hill including Elizabeth Walton, Fiona Richardson, Emma Mullenger and Astred Hicks.

Extracts from *Hospital by the River* by Dr Catherine Hamlin with John Little reprinted by permission of Pan Macmillan Australia Pty Ltd. Copyright © Dr Catherine Hamlin and John Little 2001.
For information on the Fistula Hospital, please go to <www.fistulatrust. org>. Hamlin Fistula Relief and Aid Fund, PO Box 965, Wahroonga NSW 2076. Email: fistulaltd@ozemail.com.au

Extracts from Fred Hollows' autobiography are reprinted by permission of the Fred Hollows Foundation. The Fred Hollows Foundation is a non-government organisation which seeks to eradicate avoidable blindness in developing countries and to improve the health of Indigenous Australians. Visit <www.hollows.org.au> or call 1800 352 352 to find out more.

Proceeds from the sale of this book will be donated to the Karmel Trust of Flinders University and the National Research Centre for the Prevention of Child Abuse at Monash University.

THE AUTHORS

Adjunct Associate Professor Leanne Rowe AM is a general practitioner and runs a medical practice for medical practitioners in Melbourne, Australia (www.medicalconsulting.com.au). A past chairperson of The Royal Australian College of General Practitioners, she is currently Deputy Chancellor of Monash University and serves on the boards of *beyondblue* and Medibank Private. She worked for many years as a rural doctor and has been awarded the Rose Hunt Medal from The Royal Australian College of General Practitioners and the 'Best Individual Contribution to Health Care in Australia' award from the Australian Medical Association, for her services to medicine.

Professor Michael Kidd AM is a general practitioner and the Executive Dean of the Faculty of Health Sciences at Flinders University in Adelaide, Australia. He was Professor of General Practice at the University of Sydney from 1995 to 2009 and President of The Royal Australian College of General Practitioners from 2002 to 2006. He is chair of the Australian Government's Ministerial Advisory Committee on Blood Borne Viruses and Sexually Transmissible Infections, a member of the board of the World Organization of Family Doctors (Wonca), an adviser to the World Health Organization on primary care and mental health and chair of Doctors for the Environment Australia.

Michael Kidd and Leanne Rowe have co-authored *Save Your Life and the Lives of those You Love: Your GP's 6 Step Plan for Staying Healthy Longer*, endorsed by The Royal Australian College of General Practitioners and published by Allen and Unwin in 2008.

FOREWORD

By Professor John Murtagh AM

First Do No Harm: Being a Resilient Doctor in the 21st Century is a book that challenges the medical practitioner in many ways. It is written by general practitioners, Leanne Rowe and Michael Kidd, who in recent years have been prolific authors especially in the domain of preventive medicine. They are co-authors of the recently published book 'Save your life and the lives of those you love: your GP's 6-step guide to staying healthy longer'. Predictably this book is well written and a comfortable read for both healthcare professionals and lay people. The authors have also canvassed the opinions of a range of practitioners and consumers about coping guidelines for both doctors and patients.

The book presents a subtle and clever twist to the time honoured Hippocratic tenet 'first do no harm' with the focus on doctors, their families and their patients. According to the authors 'in this book we are advocating for a broader definition of 'first do no harm' to include not just ensuring the safety of our patients but also doing no self inflicted harm' through an inappropriate professional lifestyle. They emphasise that this strategy is to facilitate building relationships at all levels including self, one's doctor, colleagues, family and friends, patients, the physical environment and medical organisations.

The authors have served The Royal Australian College of General Practitioners and their profession with distinction and are well known for their passion for special causes that are particularly significant for them. Subsequently readers will not be surprised that the text includes features on role model doctors, doctor safety, difficult patients including patient initiated violence, stress management, indigenous health and caring for the environment.

The book has a heavy emphasis on stress management which includes long lists of stressors to act as an aide memoir and also many reflective questions to challenge the reader. In fact there are many challenges to become more responsible and well balanced professionals. These include having our personal doctor, recognising our limitations, optimal time management, organising pleasant distractions such as massages, enjoying pets and special 'time out'.

It is pleasing to note that important topics such as sexuality, bullying and mindfulness, personality disorders, home visitation and conflict resolution are addressed.

The text is embellished by several high points such as the inter-action with a survivor of the *Titanic* disaster, Michael Kidd's excellent columns 'how do I know when I have had a good day' and 'message for medical students' and also profiles of iconic doctors. Other enhancements include scholarly quotations to introduce each section and boxed practice tips which contain helpful words of wisdom. Some of these tips are the original deliberations of the authors and others selected from writers such as Associate Professor Moira Sim that have caught the imagination of the authors with the theme of safe practice management in mind.

A challenging book for the thinking doctor!

CONTENTS

INTRODUCTION

If I am not for myself, who will be for me? And when I am for myself, what am 'I'? And if not now, when?

Hillel the Elder (*c.*110 BCE–10 CE), religious leader

In our time as members of the medical profession over the last 30 years, our work has been both professionally rewarding and personally challenging. We have enjoyed wonderful support from our colleagues, teachers, mentors and families. We have also learned many personal lessons, some by bitter experience. This book is about principles we now wish we had been taught about medical life and resilience before embarking on our medical careers.

One of our major life lessons has been to find balance in caring for our patients and caring for ourselves. In this book, the new meaning of the creed 'first do no harm' is not only about protecting our patients, it is also about protecting the wellbeing of our colleagues, our families, our environment and *ourselves*. Resilience is the ability to remain strong and to grow stronger when facing adversity. To remain resilient and to care for others, we must also care for ourselves. We believe that personal and peer support for doctors should not be optional.

As doctors, we carry an enormous sense of obligation and commitment to our patients. For this reason, the medical profession has had a long and admirable, but often unhealthy, tradition of self-sacrifice to work. The culture of the medical profession is such that the signs of burnout are often worn as badges of honour. It's time to change the attitude that being a stressed and miserable medical practitioner is the sign of a dedicated doctor.

There are many confusing trends confronting doctors of the 21st century. It is a paradox that more than 50% of doctors are considering leaving medical practice or reducing their hours at a time of exciting advances in medical research and innovative medical treatments. It is a tragedy that doctors have a much higher suicide rate than the general population and high levels of mental illness, yet few of us have our own doctor. It is a concern that patient satisfaction with doctors is falling and many patients seek unproven treatments in preference to consulting a doctor at a time when life expectancy of the general population is improving due to evidence-based medical interventions.

To understand these negative trends we need to step back to see how we may be inadvertently contributing to them. The tendency of doctors to be perfectionist, self-critical and risk averse are traits which can make us great doctors but which can also make us individuals with whom it can be difficult to live and difficult to work. When we raise the bar too high, it can become impossible to meet our own expectations and the result can be burnout, which can have an adverse effect on our care of our patients. When doctors are dissatisfied, patients often become dissatisfied.

While our medical organisations advise us to seek professional support and balance between our work and home life, our medical culture is not conducive to doing so. In reality, medical workplaces can be harsh environments and there seems to be very little understanding for doctors who are seen not to be carrying their weight.

As doctors, it is imperative for us to look beyond our personal horizons and to embrace a bigger story. In order to meet the new challenges facing medicine in the 21st century, effective doctors must also take time for building strong relationships and seeking peer support.

This book is for doctors of all specialties at all career stages, including medical students, recent graduates, doctors in training, experienced doctors and those approaching or beyond retirement. It's about a range of potentially harmful issues confronting doctors in everyday practice and how to address them: preventing and dealing with excessive stress; leveraging time; being proactive with our relationships with our family and friends; identifying our role models; responding to patients with challenging or confronting behaviours; dealing with criticism and complaints; caring for our own physical and mental health and dealing with personal crisis.

Most books on doctors' health and wellbeing focus on personal strategies such as the principles of cognitive behavioural therapy and on individual behaviours. While these principles have been summarised in our book, we believe that doctors require much more than individual strategies or individual counselling. We need to work together to challenge negative aspects of the culture of our profession.

This book proposes eight principles towards being a resilient doctor and these points are discussed in the final chapter:

Make home a sanctuary.
Value strong relationships.
Have an annual preventive health assessment.
Control stress, not people.
Recognise conflict as an opportunity.
Manage bullying and violence assertively.
Make our medical organisations work for us.
Create a legacy.

First Do No Harm: Being a Resilient Doctor in the 21st Century is about building strong relationships with our families, our friends, our colleagues, our patients, our medical organisations and *ourselves*.

But most of all it's about discovering and then rediscovering each day the great joy of being a doctor.

Never forget that we are privileged to be medical practitioners. Each of us makes a positive contribution to the lives of our patients every single day.

Leanne Rowe and Michael Kidd

HOW DO I KNOW WHEN I HAVE HAD A GOOD DAY IN MY PRACTICE?

- I've asked the right questions and at least one person has cried and at least one person has laughed in my consulting room.
- I've had at least one person tell me the real reason why they have come to see me.
- I've learned something new about human existence.
- I've increased my medical knowledge.
- I've cared about what happened to each patient and each colleague I have seen today.

Michael Kidd

CHAPTER 1

A NEW MEANING FOR 'FIRST DO NO HARM' IN THE 21st CENTURY

Heights by great men reached and kept were not attained by sudden flight.
They, while their fellow men slept, were toiling far into the night.

Henry Wadsworth Longfellow (1807–1882), poet and educator

The Hippocratic Oath is an example of outstanding medical leadership which has endured for more than 24 centuries. While some of the principles are more than outdated, many remain steadfast examples of how we should lead our lives as medical practitioners.

THE HIPPOCRATIC OATH

I swear by Apollo Physician and Asclepius and Hygieia and Panaceia and all the gods and goddesses, making them my witnesses, that I will fulfil according to my ability and judgment this oath and this covenant:

To hold him who has taught me this art as equal to my parents and to live my life in partnership with him, and if he is in need of money to give him a share of mine, and to regard his offspring as equal to my brothers in male lineage and to teach

them this art—if they desire to learn it—without fee and covenant; to give a share of precepts and oral instruction and all the other learning to my sons and to the sons of him who has instructed me and to pupils who have signed the covenant and have taken an oath according to the medical law, but no one else.

I will apply dietetic measures for the benefit of the sick according to my ability and judgment; I will keep them from harm and injustice.

I will neither give a deadly drug to anybody who asked for it, nor will I make a suggestion to this effect. Similarly I will not give to a woman an abortive remedy. In purity and holiness I will guard my life and my art.

I will not use the knife, not even on sufferers from stone, but will withdraw in favour of such men as are engaged in this work.

Whatever houses I may visit, I will come for the benefit of the sick, remaining free of all intentional injustice, of all mischief and in particular of sexual relations with both female and male persons, be they free or slaves.

What I may see or hear in the course of the treatment or even outside of the treatment in regard to the life of men, which on no account one must spread abroad, I will keep to myself, holding such things shameful to be spoken about.

If I fulfil this oath and do not violate it, may it be granted to me to enjoy life and art, being honoured with fame among all men for all time to come; if I transgress it and swear falsely, may the opposite of all this be my lot.[1]

Since the time of Hippocrates, the practice of medicine as a higher calling and life career has been based on high ethical standards and proud traditions. Every day doctors in every country of the world practise medicine according to a creed that has been handed down through generations: *Primum non nocere*, or 'first do no harm'.

In the opinion of some scholars, Hippocrates originated this creed in his writing on *Epidemics* in the statement 'As to diseases make a habit of two things—to help or at least to do no harm'. The creed has become an international fundamental principle to remind

1   Translation from the Greek by Ludwig Edelstein (1943), *The Hippocratic Oath: Text, Translation, and Interpretation*, Baltimore: Johns Hopkins Press.

doctors to consider possible harm to patients in every interaction and intervention. It could be argued that the creed is even more relevant in the 21st century, as many expensive technological developments in medical, surgical and pharmaceutical treatments risk increasing human suffering and can create ethical dilemmas, particularly at the end of life.

In this book, we are advocating for a broader definition of 'first do no harm', to include not just ensuring the safety of our patients but also doing no harm to ourselves. We can't be effective doctors in the long term if we neglect our own health and wellbeing. In challenging the meaning of the creed, we need to be mindful of the potential personal challenges of 21st century medicine. These new challenges include:

- New ethical issues in clinical practice related to human genomics and changes in medical technology.
- Keeping up to date with enormous advances in quality patient care.
- Dealing with health information overload.
- Meeting patient demand for early diagnosis and access to new expensive health technology.
- Balancing the pressures of being the gateway to finite health resources with the needs of our individual patients.
- Pressures associated with medical workforce shortages.
- Changes in the roles of women doctors following the significant influx of women into the medical profession over the last 50 years.
- Decreasing patient satisfaction with many aspects of medical practice.
- Increasing litigation.
- Health risks such as new infections and the impact of sedentary lifestyles.
- Escalating medical workplace violence.
- Increasing government regulation and interference in our clinical work.
- Increasing administrative demands in patient and practice record keeping and reporting.

- Meeting all the above challenges while still caring for our patients.

Even with the best intentions, we sometimes find ourselves suffering unwanted personal consequences as a result of our work as healers. It seems to be increasingly difficult to retain a commitment to being a great clinician while leading a balanced life.

BEING A DOCTOR CAN BE A RISKY BUSINESS

Being a doctor can be a health risk. There are many examples of doctors being harmed in the course of responding to the needs of their patients and there are many reasons why doctors experience high levels of burnout and mental health problems. In the past, suicide has been reported as being twice as common in male doctors and four to six times as common in female doctors than in the general population, but there are very few studies of recent trends.

Unfortunately many of us perceive asking for support from a colleague as a weakness. Yet many of us experience serious marital disharmony, mental health concerns or use excessive alcohol or other drugs. Such is the stigma attached to these issues that very little research has been conducted on the extent of the problems among medical practitioners.

We may be forced by medical registration boards to undergo supervised counselling or treatment if we are identified as being in crisis, but it is more common for us to deal with health issues by self-treatment and self-referral and miss out on vital preventive health care and mental health care. Many of us don't have our own doctor. Apparently many of us don't believe we get sick or deserve high-quality impartial health care.

On the other hand, if we are proactive about our own health and wellbeing, we are more likely to be able to provide consistent high-quality patient care. By doing so, we act in our patients' best interests in the short and long term. We participate fully in the medical workforce for longer. We set a good example for our patients and for our younger colleagues about the importance of self-care and peer support.

{ *The new meaning of 'first do no harm' includes a consideration of ourselves as well as our patients. This is not to be confused with selfishness or 'looking out for number one'. It is about a long-term obligation to our own wellbeing, health and safety, which is essential for the competent medical care of others and our optimal participation in medical life.* }

CHAPTER 2

MAKE YOUR OWN CONTRIBUTION TO A GREAT LEGACY

Example is leadership ... I don't know what your destiny will be but one thing I know. The only ones among you who will be really happy are those who have sought and found how to serve.

Albert Schweitzer (1875–1965), theologian and physician

There are many fine examples of inspirational leadership by medical practitioners throughout history. Together we have created a great legacy of healing and care through our daily work with our patients and communities.

A strong leader is usually respected for their character, capacity and sense of purpose. It is worth taking time to consider the stories of resilience and the legacies of our own medical role models, whether they be clinicians, researchers or community leaders.

Role models for medical practitioners

- Who are your role models and why?
- Write down the name of the medical role model or medical leader who most inspires you.
- Write down the characteristics of that person that you admire most.
- What are their values?
- What are your values?

It is perhaps the human experience of our medical mentors that most captures our attention. In contrast, the medical curriculum has become so dominated by science that human experience seems to have been devalued.

The damaging shift towards viewing medicine almost exclusively as a science and the devaluing of experience and human interaction was noted by Sir Andrew MacPhail as early as 1933, when he wrote: 'When a medical student must be converted into a physiologist, a physicist, a chemist, a biologist, a pharmacologist and an electrician, there is no time to make a physician of him [or her] . . . That will only happen after he [or she] has gone out in the world of sickness and suffering.'

In this chapter we honour the stories of medical role models who have had a profound influence on our clinical lives; medical practitioners who wrote about their personal experiences of sickness and suffering, remained resilient in the face of adversity and left lasting legacies through their clinical work and their advocacy.

DR CATHERINE HAMLIN
AC (1924–)

We're giving a beautiful woman a new life and this is why I stay in Ethiopia.
I love them.

Dr Catherine Hamlin with **John Little**, *Hospital by the River*

Gynaecologists Catherine and Reg Hamlin left Australia in 1959 to establish a midwifery school in Ethiopia. They went on to establish the Addis Ababa Fistula Hospital and have successfully operated on more than 34 000 women. They have also advocated at an international level for funding to improve the access of women of all backgrounds and all religions, to fistula repair.

Dr Reg Hamlin would describe the suffering of women with untreated fistula:[1]

> Mourning the stillbirth of their only child, incontinent of urine, ashamed of their
> offensiveness, often spurned by their husbands, homeless, unemployable, except
> in the fields, they endure, they exist, without friends, without hope.
> They bear their sorrows in silent shame. Their miseries, untreated, are utter,
> lonely and lifelong.

Since Dr Reg Hamlin died in 1993, Dr Catherine Hamlin has continued to pioneer and teach procedures for obstetric fistula repair to surgeons from around the world. She has also opened other hospitals in other Ethiopian cities and hopes to do more about preventing birth trauma by putting a midwife in every village. Many of her accomplishments have been achieved during times of war in Ethiopia.

In a tribute to her late husband, Dr Catherine Hamlin said:

> Reg was terribly touched by the plight of these poor women. He called them the
> fistula pilgrims on account of the tremendous journeys they undertook to get to
> the capital. He would hear how they had suffered and been rejected, and of their
> struggle to get to the hospital, how they perhaps had to sell an animal or beg to
> raise the money, and often, as he listened to their stories, he would have tears in
> his eyes. If fistula sufferers turned up at outpatients, the other women would push
> them to the end of the line because they were so offensive to be near. Reg would go
> to them and put his arms around them and say, 'You're the most important patient
> to me today. I'm going to see you first.' With the fistula pilgrims he found the great
> cause he had been seeking. He was drawn to them because he loved them.
> We found that looking after them was never a hardship and never once did we
> feel we wanted to do something else.

After her husband died, Dr Catherine Hamlin found the will to continue her work through the support of her devoted staff and the inspirational stories of her patients. In her book, *The Hospital by the*

---

1 Extracts in this section are taken from Dr Catherine Hamlin with John Little (2001), *Hospital by the River*, reprinted by permission of Pan Macmillan Australia Pty Ltd, Sydney. Copyright © Dr Catherine Hamlin and John Little 2001.

River, Dr Catherine Hamlin reflected on her motivation to continue her work:

We cured so many thousands of women that most of them have become a blur. When I reflect back over the years, however, certain faces come swimming unbidden out of the tide of memory. Even though everyone's story was amazing, some were even more so. Once a young woman arrived at the hospital and handed us an envelope with a letter inside that had been written by a missionary doctor down near the Kenyan border. It introduced her and asked us to treat her fistula. There was nothing especially unusual about her. Like so many of our patients she was dressed in rags and weak from hunger. The sealed envelope was so worn and grubby you could hardly read it, but inside the clean letter was legible enough. To our surprise it had been dated seven years ago. 'Why has it taken you seven years to get here?' I asked. She told me she had been begging at the bus station for her fare. That was how long it took her to raise the money.

As I look back over my life with Reg and our work with the women of Ethiopia it surprises me sometimes to realise that I am 77 years old. Never for a moment have I felt like retiring, or wanted to change my life or my work. I still operate several times a week, and my hands are as steady as ever. Although my life has been spent working for fistula patients, the fascination and appeal has never paled.

Dr Catherine Hamlin has been made a Companion of the Order of Australia, was awarded the ANZAC Peace Prize, received the Gold Medal from the Royal College of Surgeons and was nominated for the Nobel Peace Prize.

SIR EDWARD (WEARY) DUNLOP
AC CMG OBE (1907–1993)

I have a conviction that it's only when you are put at full stretch that you can realise your full potential.

E.E. Dunlop, *The War Diaries of Weary Dunlop*

The stories of determination of doctors to provide care for their patients under the most dire situations are shining examples of medical heroism. One of the best-known examples is that of Sir Edward Dunlop.

During World War II, Sir Edward Dunlop developed a mobile surgical unit in the Middle East. After he served in Tobruk in North Africa, his troopship was diverted to Java where he was promoted to lieutenant-colonel.

In 1942 he became a prisoner of war when his hospital in Bandung, Java, was captured. In recognition of his leadership skills he was placed in charge of prisoner of war camps in Java and then commanded the Australian prisoners sent to work on the Burma–Thailand Railway in 1943.

When Sir Edward Dunlop finally returned home from the prison camps, he brought with him his medical diary, which was a unique record of the lives of prisoners of war from 1942 to 1945 and which was published more than 40 years later. Sir Edward's book describing epidemics of cholera and malaria, surgical operations in impossible conditions, torture and death raised the awareness of the Australian community to the gradual decline in pension benefits available to past prisoners of war. In the book, he said:

Of some 22 000 who entered captivity, more than 7000 died or were killed. Of their sufferings ... only those who were present can fully comprehend the seeming hopelessness of it all as their bodies wasted and their friends died ... In suffering we are all equal. [2]

In a tribute to Sir Edward, Australian writer Donald Stuart wrote:

We built a railway from near Bangkok to near Rangoon ... thousands of us Prisoners of War ... starved, scourged, racked with malaria, dysentery, beri beri, pellagra, and the stinking tropical ulcers that ate a leg to the bone ... when despair and death reached for us [Dunlop] stood fast, a lighthouse of sanity in a universe of madness and suffering.

---

2 Extracts in this section are taken from E.E. Dunlop (1986), *The War Diaries of Weary Dunlop*, Melbourne: Nation Publishers.

Fellow prisoner of war Sir Laurens van der Post described Sir Edward's leadership through these dark days:

I only know that I have the testimony of hundreds of Australians who had served with me and accompanied Weary to Burma and Siam that he was both the inspiration and the main instrument of their physical and spiritual survival. I know, moreover, from the letters I get every year from the rapidly diminishing number of those who shared our prison experience, that the memory of unique service Weary performed for them all remains with them, as it does for me, as though it were not something in the past but a forever 'now' in our beings.

Sir Edward's last entry on 16 August 1945 in his diary reflects his resilience:

This has been a war against monstrous things, but one for which we all share responsibility because of the selfish preoccupations which allowed matters to reach such hideous proportions. There will be an enduring bonus for all of us in the deep affection and comradeship which has evolved, not only between we Australians, but with men of several nations who have shared this long dark night of captivity. There will be strenuous and exciting days working to get the last of these maimed and damaged men on their way home. I have resolved to make their care and welfare a life long mission.

After the war, Sir Edward devoted himself to the health of former prisoners of war and their families. His tireless community work had a great influence in Australia and in Asia and he was later honoured by Thailand, India, Sri Lanka and the United Kingdom.

After Sir Edward died on 2 July 1993, Australia's former Governor-General Sir Zelman Cowan described Sir Edward's state funeral in these words: 'The experience . . . was altogether remarkable and it is surely one which will remain in the collective life of the nation as a celebration of human worth.'

Sir Edward Weary Dunlop has come to symbolise the work of many doctors who served their nations in times of peril. There are many who never returned home and whose stories will never be told.

PROFESSOR FRED HOLLOWS AC
(1929–1993)

You don't need to be a surgeon to restore someone's sight. It's a simple operation.

Fred Hollows with **Peter Corris**, *An Autobiography*

The author Thomas Keneally once referred to Professor Fred Hollows as 'the wild colonial boy of Australian surgery'. Through his leadership, the vision of more than one million people in Australia and developing countries has been restored. As examples of his inspirational work, he pioneered modern cataract surgery in developing countries and headed the National Trachoma and Eye Health Program in Australia, which screened the vision of 100 000 people in over 460 communities and treated more than 27 000 people for trachoma.

In his autobiography Professor Hollows reflected on the recognition of his work:[3]

In recent years I've gathered a few honours—Companion of the Order of Australia, the 1990 Australian Human Rights medal, the 1991 Humanist of the Year award, several honorary degrees and the Australian of the Year award for 1990. I've been surprised by the amount of personal gratification these gongs have given me. No one is without vanity. But accepting them has also given me a platform from which to speak out about the things that concern me—Aboriginal health and the social and political position of Aborigines, and the responsibility we, as privileged citizens of First World countries, bear to the people of the Third World. To my mind, having care and concern for others is the highest of the human qualities.

3   Extracts in this section are taken from F. Hollows with Peter Corris (1991), *An Autobiography*, Sydney: John Kerr Publishers Pty Ltd.

Before his death in 1993, he worked with his wife Gabi Hollows and his supporters to set up the Fred Hollows Foundation to ensure that his work would endure. He was honoured by a state funeral and, in keeping with his own wish, was buried in the Bourke outback. A plaque on his grave reads: 'The key he used to undo locks was vision for the poor.'

Perhaps we can learn most from his reflection on who he was and what he believed in:

I am a humanist; I don't believe in any higher power than the best expressions of the human spirit, and those are to be found in personal and social relationships. Evaluating my own life in those terms, I've had some mixed results. I've hurt some people and disappointed others but I hope that, on balance, I've given more than I've taken. I believe that my view of what 'a redeemed social condition' is has been consistent—equity between people—and I've always tried to work to that end.

I call myself an eye doctor, but casting around for another word to describe my life's work, I am reminded of my teacher's question put so long ago: 'Well Hollows, what sort of an engineer do you want to be?' The Macquarie Dictionary lists seven meanings for the word engineer. The sixth is of particular interest to me—'U.S. an engine driver', my father's honourable calling; but I am also attracted to the seventh meaning: 'to arrange, manage or carry through by skilful or artful contrivance'.

DR KHULOD MAAROUF-HASSAN
(1955–2006)

For Dr Maarouf-Hassan, being a doctor was very natural. It was in her being.

A patient

Dr Khulod Maarouf-Hassan's story was one of quiet perseverance through adversity. She was born in Syria, and graduated from medical school in 1978. As well as completing her training as an ophthalmologist, she had a passion for mathematics, Arabic literature and politics. After she emigrated to Australia with her husband in 1986, she was unable to become registered as a doctor and worked for about 10 years in a milk bar. In 1999 Dr Maarouf-Hassan passed the medical entry examination and she entered the Australian General Practice Training Program. After a long journey, Dr Maarouf-Hassan was awarded the Fellowship of the Royal Australian College of General Practitioners in 2005.

Dr Maarouf-Hassan chose to work in disadvantaged communities; to carry on the proud tradition of her family. She was passionate about assisting refugees in her general practice. Her daughter Nawaar says she stopped asking her mother why she was arriving home so late from work, after she replied: 'One family walked 4 hours to see me. How could I turn them away?'.

On 16 June 2006, an ex-patient entered her general practice during office hours and without any warning brutally stabbed Dr Maarouf-Hassan to death. This acutely psychotic man had pleaded for help from many organisations for protection from members of the whole medical profession who he believed were trying to kill him. Tragically, no one responded to his pleas for help. To this day, no one understands why this young man chose Dr Maarouf-Hassan as his victim as he had only consulted her twice, nine months before her death. In the words of the prosecution lawyer in the Supreme Court trial, 'She could not have done more as a doctor. She could not have cared more for her patients.'

The collective grief of the Australian medical profession and the Australian community following this tragedy was palpable. The news of this quiet achiever's death was international news. More than 2000 people attended her funeral in a simple community hall. Perhaps the most poignant tribute came from one of her patients:

The more I think what kind of person Dr Maarouf has been, the more I realise there are no words to express it. First of all I just want to say that she has been the kind of doctor, despite her greatness, [who] makes you feel very important, puts you at ease, and makes you feel very comfortable and safe. She just had this inner conviction that she genuinely cares. And it takes a lot for me to trust someone, and the more I knew her the more I trusted her. She was very generous with her time. Personally, she is my hero and I'm very grateful to Dr Maarouf for everything. And I can only hope that she's going to make such a great difference in people's lives through her death. So thank you, thank you to Dr Maarouf, and her family for sharing her with us.

More than one million Australians watched the 2008 TV program *Australian Story* on Dr Maarouf-Hassan's life and death. In the words of one viewer:

I would have loved to have known Khulod—and had such a wonderful doctor. She was a great Australian, she was a dedicated doctor committed to helping the underprivileged, a loving and supportive wife. A devoted and caring mother and friend to her children. In all things, putting others first. But it is not only her family that has lost this special woman. It is also the greater community's loss that she is no longer physically with us. Her legacy will live on through her three young daughters.

These stories inspire thought about the characteristics of courageous medical practitioners including the somewhat paradoxical combination of fierce determination and humility. In their autobiographies, these doctors admit to feeling fear and frustration, facing failure and being human. What they have in common is the ability to meet everyday and extraordinary challenges and to recognise adversity as an opportunity to grow and to make a meaningful contribution. As well as inner strength, resolve and determination, they share a sense of humour and the ability to laugh at their own foibles. These are qualities shared by many medical practitioners working with their local communities all around the world.

If you believe in yourself, you can move mountains and fill in the ocean; no matter how difficult the task, you will see the day when you succeed.

Dr Sun Yat-Sen, (1866–1925) Hong Kong General Practitioner, and later Chinese Revolutionary Leader

Resilience

- Who or what inspires you after a challenging experience?
- When your heart sinks or your eyes fill with tears, what is it that lifts your spirits again?

Try writing about those unforgettable encounters when you are faced with the overwhelming evidence of the value of your work.

Medical practitioners at all stages of their careers and especially our more senior colleagues can share their stories in a way that inspires future generations of doctors.

Too often we hear of doctors saying 'how much worse things were in their day' to younger colleagues. It is important to embrace a bigger story about our lives as doctors. Seldom have an inventory of personal beliefs and a sense of values underpinning our work been more needed to sustain us.

Your journal

Many great writers have also been doctors and observers of human nature and through their writing shared their reflections. Just think of Aristotle, Keats, Chekhov, Somerset Maugham and Sir Arthur Conan Doyle. Consider keeping a journal or notebook of your own observations, your insights into humanity, your patients' letters and your reflections on your mentors, your teachers and your work. It will become a priceless collection of your individual contribution as an extraordinary doctor.

As medical practitioners we are part of a great legacy of caring for other people. Through our individual actions we can each make our own lasting contribution to this great shared legacy to humankind.

CHAPTER 3

ON BEING A DOCTOR

*This is the true joy in life: Being used for a purpose recognized by yourself as
a mighty one, being a force of nature instead of a feverish, selfish little clod of
ailments and grievances, complaining that the world will not devote itself to making
you happy. I am of the opinion that my life belongs to the whole community and as
long as I live, it is my privilege to do for it what I can. It is a sort of splendid torch
which I have got hold of for the moment and I want to make it burn as brightly as
possible before handing it on to future generations.*

George Bernard Shaw (1856–1950), playwright

Many of us chose medicine as a career so that we could make
a difference to the wellbeing of people and communities.
Medicine is a rewarding career. But as with any challenging work,
the reality of a medical career can be demanding, consuming and
uncertain. In this book, we advocate taking the time to plan our
medical and personal lives just as we plan for the ongoing training in
our clinical work.

The community has very high expectations of its doctors as
care providers and community leaders. Doctors are expected, and
we expect ourselves, to be always competent, caring, concerned,
responsible, sensitive, trustworthy and honest. The internal pressure
constantly to maintain these qualities can be exhausting, particularly
at a time of chronic medical workforce shortage.

Most books concerning the health of doctors begin with the
problems associated with our driven personalities and the advantages
of adopting a more relaxed approach. While the Type A/B personality
theory has been recently questioned as oversimplistic, many of us
continue to identify strongly with these characteristics.

MESSAGE FOR MEDICAL STUDENTS

As you begin your career, stop and consider 'What sort of a doctor am I going to be?'.

If you are going to be a great doctor, throughout your studies and throughout your career you will need to:

- retain your common sense;
- retain your good humour;
- retain your sense of humility;
- retain your commitment to being a great clinician; and
- lead a balanced life.

Michael Kidd

Many of us tend to develop driven personalities in order to meet the excessive demands of medical life and to get the job done. In this situation, a driven personality should be seen as a useful adaptation rather than a weakness or personality flaw. However, problems can arise when we bring some of these personality traits into our personal lives. Sometimes it can be hard to live and work with us. Consider these characteristics of a driven personality which make many of us great doctors but perhaps also somewhat difficult and challenging individuals.

THE DRIVEN PERSONALITY

Recognising a driven personality

- Are you very irritable when late?
  Are you often late because of unexpected emergencies and long consultations and increasing patient demand?

- Are you impatient while waiting?
  Do you get frustrated, thinking that you will run even later if you have to wait for others?
- Are you a fast eater?
  Have you been conditioned to eat quickly or risk not eating at all?
- Are you a hard task master?
  Do you have an endless 'to do list' but also expect to achieve balance between your work and home lives?
- Are you interested in very little outside home and work?
  Do you find that you have very little personal social time because when you are not at work you are making up for lost time with your family responsibilities? Is alcohol, including wine appreciation, one of your only hobbies?
- Are you very competitive and ambitious?
  Were you encouraged to compete during student years for rankings and later for postgraduate training positions?
- Are you someone who anticipates what others are going to say and sometimes finish their sentences?
  Are you a highly intuitive active listener, experienced with interpreting body language, but sometimes frustrated with how long it takes for others to express their thoughts?
- Are you always in a rush?
  Do you receive complaints if you keep patients waiting or if your appointments are booked out for weeks ahead? Does the threat of medico-legal action hang over your practice and lead you to double-check everything you do? Do you find it a challenge accommodating patients who present with urgent medical problems, but at the same time feel pressured to make adequate time available for review of your current patients?
- Are you trying to do too many things at once, and at the same time thinking about what you will do next?
  Do you find it a challenge constantly pre-empting problems, assessing risks, managing multiple problems and having to make complex decisions?

- Are you seeking to be recognised by others?
  Do you find you rarely receive recognition because patients, family and friends expect you to maintain your caring role outside your work and rarely give you positive feedback because they assume you know you are appreciated?

- Are you someone who hides your feelings?
  Do you put your own feelings on hold while you empathise with patients or attend to the medical task at hand?

- Are you someone who feels guilty when doing nothing?
  Are you accustomed to having free time? Or does someone always manage to find something for you to do? Do you find it difficult to say no?

- Are you never really happy?
  Do you have a perfectionist, self-critical personality? Do you have a harsh inner voice? Have you set the bar too high? Do you think in terms of 'I must', 'I should' or 'I always'? Is this how you have been taught to think about clinical decision making as a medical student?

- Are you someone who gets satisfaction only when results are achieved?
  Do you find leaving unfinished work is not an option because you have been trained to treat health problems decisively and thoroughly?

Overwork is often seen as the sign of a dedicated doctor. Those of us who have the characteristics of driven personalities are often rewarded professionally and financially. We receive few complaints, rarely make mistakes and are conscientious and dedicated. We complete most of our tasks by the due date, constantly pre-empt problems, manage risks and work long hours to go beyond what is expected of us.

Many of these personality traits are important to get the job done. But when as doctors we become task orientated and slaves to endless 'to do lists' at the expense of our relationships, our lives can start to fall apart.

NEGATIVE STRESS

Many of us enjoy the mental challenge of positive stress. For example, having to react quickly and competently in emergency situations or manage complex medical dilemmas is often rewarding and satisfying. Negative stress is very different and is often defined as an imbalance between perceived demand and the perception of one's ability to meet that demand. At its heart, negative stress is fundamentally about perceived loss of control. In medical practice, the external demands and flow of information are often excessive. Change is stressful yet medicine is constantly changing. It is often impossible to meet all the demands. It is realistic to feel, at times, as if things are out of our control.

Negative stress can be associated with common life events including transition to work from university, marriage, becoming a parent, illness or death in a family member or friend, separation and divorce, retirement, problems with sexual relationships, change in business or financial status, taking on a mortgage or loan, conflict with extended family, moving house or clinic or even the holiday season. These life events can cause anyone to become stressed. In addition to these stressors, as doctors we must juggle many other causes of stress in medical practice. It's worth taking time to identify sources and symptoms of stress.

OUR STRESS BUCKET

As one of the major causes of feeling stressed is a sense of feeling out of control, we need to identify the causes of stress we can control, rather than trying to influence things we have no control over.

Your stress bucket

Think of yourself as a stress bucket. It can help to list all the stresses that fill your bucket and recognise the signs that let you know when your stress bucket is overflowing.

☞

☞

Use the following headings:
Signs of your full bucket (signs of stress)
Causes of your full bucket (sources of stress)
Ways to release your full bucket (solutions to stress)

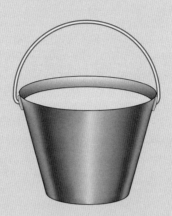

If you would like to explore this in more detail, on the left side of a page list all the times and situations when you have felt stressed over the past few days, and on the right side try to answer these questions:

- What did you think, do or try when you felt stressed?
- Did it help?
- What could you have done differently?
- What may help next time?
- What were the circumstances beyond your control?
- What were the circumstances within your control?
- What can you do about them?
- Where can you seek support?
- Imagine that your problem has been solved; how would you feel?
- How would you know this had happened?

By using these exercises and drawing on past challenging experiences, we can discover that adversity is an opportunity to learn from mistakes, to grow and to enrich our lives. In the next chapter we will discuss ways to release the pressure in the stress bucket in more detail.

SIGNS OF STRESS

Here are some of the well-known *short-term signs* of excessive stress:

- Dry mouth
- Muscle tension
- Sweating
- Palpitations
- Breathlessness

The *longer-term signs* of stress can include:

- Feelings of quiet desperation and being unable to cope
- Feelings of helplessness or hopelessness
- Worrying excessively and unreasonably about things outside our control or things that have not happened yet
- Frustration, irritability and pent up anger
- Intolerance of minor problems or transgressions by other people
- Excessive mood swings
- Withdrawing into daydreams
- Apathy and feeling tired all the time
- Compassion fatigue or inability to feel sympathy for others
- Tearfulness and sadness
- Indecisiveness and being prone to mistakes
- Inefficiency, doing many things at once and always being rushed
- Resistance to change or inflexibility
- Lack of interest in leisure pursuits or self-appearance
- Change in eating habits including bingeing or skipping meals
- Physical symptoms such as headache, backache, neck ache, indigestion, irritable bowel or excessive health concerns
- Anxiety and depression

Burnout is related to chronic stress and may be related to chronic physical health problems, relationship problems, entrenched negative thinking and risky behaviours.

SOURCES OF STRESS

Here are some of the issues that some of our colleagues have nominated as their major sources of stress.

ATTITUDES

- Lack of acknowledgment of our work
- Patient anger at their diagnosis or the failure of treatment recommendations
- Lack of patient understanding when their doctor is sick
- Increasing anti-doctor sentiment in the community and in the media

TIME PRESSURE

- Coping with excessive numbers of phone calls, repeated interruptions
- Emergency calls, after-hours calls and unrelenting long hours of work
- Financial pressures which may cause doctors to rush patients to generate more income
- Pressure to see more and more patients due to the medical workforce shortage

UNREALISTIC EXPECTATIONS

- Increasing community expectations and patient dissatisfaction
- Complaints about long waiting times and waiting lists
- Constant need to show empathy
- Dealing with expectations by friends and relatives to be their carer
- The expectation that full-time doctors will consult with hundreds of patients each week

- The monotony of repetitive tasks
- The expectation to work past the age when many other professional people retire

LACK OF WORKPLACE SUPPORT

- Poor remuneration for some medical specialties, especially in lower socioeconomic areas
- Costs of setting up and maintaining a medical practice
- Lack of adequate support from the wider health system for patients with mental health and drug and alcohol problems
- Occupational hazards including risk of exposure to serious infections
- Difficulty in negotiating employment contracts
- Separation from family during medical training
- Professional isolation especially in rural areas
- Lack of access and planning for sick leave, annual leave and long-service leave
- Lack of training about the business side of medical practice
- Administrative overload and the demands of bureaucratic paperwork
- Inexperienced members of staff and feeling that there is inadequate time to train new people properly
- Conflict with practice partners and with other staff in the practice or hospital
- Competition with neighbouring practices
- Problems with the physical environment of the hospital or practice including excessive noise, lack of car parking, poor cooling and heating, fluorescent lighting, poorly designed workspaces
- Government interference in clinical independence

LACK OF WORK—FAMILY BALANCE

- Feelings of lack of personal control due to inflexibility of workload
- Effect of demands of work on family time

- Lack of emotional support at home from partner and the inability to provide emotional support at home for partner and children
- Distant relationships with children and the inability to share parenting tasks
- Chronic sleep deprivation
- Unsatisfactory or no social life
- Challenge of locating suitable child care arrangements

PATIENT CARE ISSUES

- Daily contact with people who are suffering
- 'Therapeutic impotence'—being unable to treat some serious disorders
- Fear of making mistakes and threat of litigation
- Dealing with uncertainty in diagnosis and management
- Ethical dilemmas in patient care
- Risk of physical and verbal assault by patients

TRAINING AND PROFESSIONAL COMPETENCY ISSUES

- Choosing an area of medical specialty and career path
- Professional activities such as professional development, quality assurance and practice accreditation, all of which take time

GROUPS OF DOCTORS MORE AT RISK

There are certain times in each doctor's career when stress is more likely to be a problem. And there are certain features of different groups of doctors which may lead to different types of stress.

NEW DOCTORS

The time of transition from medical student to intern can be a time of great excitement but also one of serious stress for many new doctors. New doctors report many stresses including meeting the demands and expectations of senior colleagues, learning to work with other health professionals and other hospital staff, feeling undervalued and coping with the stress of working long hours, night shifts and after hours.

Some new doctors find it difficult to balance the demands of work and family and friends and also experience the significant pressures of having to prepare for specialist training assessments. Junior doctors often feel overwhelmed when confronted with large numbers of patients and what may be seen as unrealistic patient expectations. Some feel overwhelmed by the responsibility of patient care. The sudden realisation that the 'buck stops here' can be daunting. Many new doctors benefit from seeking mentorship or professional support from more senior colleagues.

WOMEN DOCTORS

Women doctors commonly experience more constraints on their career ambitions and more concerns about effects of work on family life. Many women continue to perform traditional roles of daughter, wife and mother as well as meet their professional responsibilities.

Career options may be limited by the need to take time out of training for childbirth and child rearing. There can be challenges maintaining competence while working part-time. Family commitments are often undervalued by colleagues. In the past there have been fewer senior women role models to emulate. Women are more likely to experience discrimination and violence in the workplace.

RURAL DOCTORS

Rural doctors tend to find it more difficult to obtain locum and peer support. In rural areas there is often more after-hours work and less access to training and specialist support. Rural doctors are more likely to feel isolated and at times out of their depth. Their families often bear the brunt of these stresses and their children are often sent away for education. Professional boundaries are more difficult to maintain for doctors working and living in rural areas.

DOCTORS EMIGRATING TO A NEW COUNTRY

Doctors moving to a new country face multiple stresses including the stress of change for themselves and their families, the need to engage in further training and study in order to have their qualifications recognised, the lack of available support from extended family members and community, the lack of engagement with a peer group of colleagues, professional isolation if required to practise in remote locations, and the stress of being separated from partner and children if the doctor has emigrated first. There is also stress associated with cultural change and lack of awareness of local cultural norms.

AGEING DOCTORS

Older doctors can be a great source of wisdom and advice to younger colleagues about how to build resilience and manage the many stresses of a busy life as a clinician. Many of us gain great support through having an older, more experienced colleague as a mentor.

Many doctors continue to work beyond the age when their peers retire. Worldwide workforce shortages are demanding that they remain in clinical practice. Many doctors feel under pressure to continue to work full-time in clinical practice in order to meet financial commitments, especially related to practice and insurance costs and the desire to provide for their family members.

Retirement itself can be a time of stressful life change as previously busy people find themselves with time on their hands, without a sense of purpose and socially isolated.

Many ageing doctors continue to work even if they themselves are experiencing the effects of chronic disease, chronic pain or mental health concerns. Many doctors fail to seek or heed the advice that they might give their own patients about slowing down, considering retirement, engaging in other worthwhile pursuits and enjoying many of the joys of the later years of life.

THE STRESS WE CREATE FOR OURSELVES

One of the strategies for treating depression is to raise our patients' awareness of their assertive rights and the assertive rights of others. Along with other cognitive behavioural therapy strategies, people with depression are often advised to practise repeating their personal rights, which may include the following:[1]

- I have the right to be the judge of what I do and what I think.
- I have the right to offer no reasons or excuses for my behaviour.
- I have the right to refuse to be responsible for finding solutions to other people's problems.
- I have the right to change my mind.
- I have the right to make mistakes.
- I have the right to say I don't know.
- I have the right to make my own decisions.
- I have the right to say I don't understand.
- I have the right to say I don't care.
- I have the right to say no without feeling guilty.

This list exposes the difference between the assertive rights of patients and the assertive rights of doctors. While these personal rights seem reasonable for the rest of the community, many of them can be difficult for doctors to assert during their professional work. In fact, a meeting with the local Medical Practitioners' Board would be in order if statements like these were used inappropriately by a doctor in a consultation with a patient. This does not mean that as doctors we cannot assert our own rights in our relationships with our patients. We compensate for not being able to assert some of these rights by creating space and boundaries in our relationships with our patients.

While time for solitude is often helpful, prolonged isolation will fail to rejuvenate us and may be destructive. The reaction to symptoms of stress may be to withdraw from other people as it is common to feel as though we have nothing left to give after a challenging day's work. However distancing ourselves from other people, especially our main supports, can begin a spiral of increasing problems including depression and excessive alcohol use.

---

1   Treatment Protocol Project (2004), *Management of Mental Disorder*, 4th edn, Sydney: World Health Organization, Collaborating Centre for Evidence in Mental Health Policy.

Sometimes as doctors, we may ruminate about our sense of responsibility and we may even experience a sense of martyrdom. Putting in 100% effort 100% of the time is exhausting, and the self-expectation *to be everything to everyone all of the time* can lead to an exaggerated sense of responsibility. Many of us are overconscientious and work harder to satisfy a need for status or to resolve feelings of self-doubt or an unconscious fear of failure. Many high achievers never feel perfect enough. It is very tiring to try to anticipate other's needs constantly and to pre-empt all risks. It's easy to become emotionally detached when there is no outlet for painful emotions.

As doctors we may find we use work as an excuse and a defence. The competitive urge for a better job, higher status and greater income can be stressful.

We risk blaming work rather than taking an active approach to identifying stressors and stepping back to solve them. It is worth thinking about how we may create unnecessary distress by failing to meet our own impossible expectations and failing to seek personal support.

> *Even driven people have their limits. If we are going to be effective clinicians we need to recognise the warning signs of stress and make changes in our lives to restore a sense of balance. Most of the time we know the right things to do but we delay making decisions and don't actually get around to doing what we need to do to help ourselves. Sometimes the greatest challenge is just getting us to put into place what we already know we should be doing.*

CHAPTER 4

OUR RELATIONSHIP WITH OURSELVES

*To regard states of distress in general as an objection, as something that must
be abolished, is the supreme idiocy, in a general sense a real disaster in its
consequences…almost as stupid as the will to abolish bad weather.*

Friedrich Nietzsche (1844–1900), philosopher

Dealing with excessive demands is a normal part of being a doctor.
For this reason, it is important to be honest with ourselves, to
seek support when we need to, to identify areas where we may not be
strong and to look after our minds and bodies.

OUR SPIRITUAL AND EMOTIONAL HEALTH

Our spiritual and emotional health are enhanced by spending
time with people who inspire and energise us, by being involved
in creative and uplifting pastimes and by reflecting on and valuing
challenging experiences and personal strengths. But from very early
in our careers doctors are taught the necessity of self-denial while
dealing with the tasks at hand and delaying gratification. There is a
risk that we may accept life as a state of chronic stress.

Sometimes we strive to be free of stress, but forget to aim for wellbeing. We can forget what feeling normal is like. When we feel well, our minds feel balanced and our physical health improves.

But improving our wellbeing is easier said than done when there is never enough time and it can be difficult to maintain a proactive approach to our spiritual, emotional and physical health. At times of heavy workload and sleep deprivation it can be easy to slip into negative rumination, self-criticism, bad temper, self-absorption and self-doubt, which are very destructive.

In our society, the preoccupation with personal happiness based on consumerism, materialism, perceived status and escapism can be enticing. Most of us know life satisfaction and contentment come from having a greater goal or cause than oneself. Finding meaning in work, physical and emotional closeness with others, joy in living and an appreciation of the miracle and mystery of life are all part of feeling alive as a human being. Resilience comes from transcending challenges by focusing on bigger goals and valuing our relationships.

Emotional intelligence is about self-control and self-mastery and the ability to get on with oneself and others. It's about feeling, understanding and using emotions positively. By being in touch with our emotions and using them productively, we can in turn work productively with other people and their emotions. In this chapter we raise some questions which help us reflect on our emotional intelligence and we discuss some alternative ways to respond to excessive stress.

Interview yourself

Consider a popular job interview question: 'Describe how you worked through a major challenge.'

While it is tempting to impress interviewers with a story of individual success, instead describe a major challenge where, despite your best efforts, no resolution was found, but important life lessons were learned and other people were acknowledged. Learning from such events can be important steps in our maturation as clinical leaders.

OUR PURPOSE

A mighty purpose gives us strength to endure adversity. It gives us meaning for living and working and helps us overcome temporary setbacks. Having clear goals in all areas of our lives will help us maintain an optimistic outlook. It can be helpful to reflect on our goals regularly to ensure we know what we really want from life, why our goals are important, what our values and priorities are and how we are travelling.

Your purpose

Consider your response to each of these questions:
* What is the mighty purpose of your life?
* What are your goals now and how will they help you achieve your life purpose?
* Why is each of your current goals important?
* What are your priorities?
* What were your goals in the past and have you achieved these?
* If not, why not?

A life purpose is an overarching statement about what inspires us. It tends not to change with time. Goals help us achieve our purpose and may change over time. Setting goals can be a very difficult exercise. If this is the case, we can try breaking down our goals in different aspects of our lives.

Where are you going?

You might like to try answering any of the following questions which are of interest to you.

Your spiritual life

Who or what inspires you? What are your beliefs? What is your purpose? What do you find uplifting? What are your values? What legacy would you like to contribute to? What are you passionate about?

Other people

Which relationships are most important to you? What qualities do you seek in your relationships?

Your home

How can you make your home a sanctuary from the challenges of your work life?

Your physical health

How can you fit exercise into your daily life? How will you approach preventive health care?

Your medical career

What are your short-term career goals? What are your long-term career goals? What is your plan for lifelong learning? What are your goals for the development of your professional career over the next 12 months? Or the next five years?

Your financial situation

What is your financial plan? How much money is enough? What do you need to do in the short term and the long term? Have you obtained competent advice? Do you have adequate insurance?

Your social and personal life

What social activities energise you and give you the greatest pleasure? What places would you like to visit? Where are you planning your holidays over the next 12 months? Have you planned a period of long-service leave of at least three months at least once every 10 years?

Finally, you might like to consider the following:

- What are your clear and achievable realistic goals for the next few months?
- What do you wish to achieve in each area of your life during the coming 5 to 10 years?
- What is your plan for how to achieve your goals in the next 5 or 10 years?

Sometimes we set goals and then find it difficult to implement them.

Here are some questions that may help reflect on common sources of frustration and why it is often difficult to achieve our goals. We don't have to deal with all the stressors but it may help to identify our priorities and to deal with those issues first.

Challenge yourself

Identify which of the following questions resonate for you. Tick the questions you think may help you challenge yourself.

☐ What are the best and worst things about your work?

☐ What are the top three frustrations of your work?

☐ What advice would you give to a new colleague or a son or daughter going into medical practice?

☐ What are the greatest barriers to your practice of good medicine?

☐ What do you want to get from your work?

☐ What are the ways to make this happen?

☐ Are there things you would like to be doing that you're not doing?

☐ What changes would you like to see in your life?

☐ Where should your priorities be?

☐ If you had a magic wand, what would you most change at work and home?

☐ What can you do now to improve your work and life balance?

☐ Which people and what situations get under your skin? Why?

☐ Why, how and where are you spending your time?

☐ What would you like to do more of?

☐ What can you delegate, safely avoid or defer?

☐ Imagine you could actually have everything you wanted. What would you do differently and can you do that now?

☐ Are you happy?

DEALING WITH ISSUES IN OUR CONTROL

In the last chapter we discussed the concept of the stress bucket. Here are some ways some of our colleagues have recommended to try to relieve the pressure in our own stress buckets.

PATIENT CARE

- Plan ahead to allow regular breaks throughout the day at work and throughout the year.
- Maintain professional boundaries at work and outside work. For example, avoid discussing medical issues with patients and other people away from the workplace.
- Remember to seek joy in relationships with patients by sharing their achievements, stories of courage and wisdom, pride in their children and grandchildren. Doctors can gain deep insights into life by doing so.

ACHIEVE WORK—LIFE BALANCE

- Live near loved ones if at all possible.
- Make home a sanctuary by listening to family members' needs and taking time to relax with them.
- Speak to a confidante regularly; try not to store worries, unload them.
- Practise regular meditation, mindfulness, relaxation techniques, music therapy or writing therapy.
- Take time to switch off every day.
- Make time for solo time and take time out for solitude.
- Have a regular massage.
- Slow down whenever possible.
- Practise slow breathing when standing in a queue or sitting in a traffic jam.
- Eat slowly and enjoy each meal. Healthy nutrition takes time.
- Take regular time off and engage in some social activities that are not competitive. Develop interests outside medicine. To make up for a sedentary day job consider bushwalking, surfing,

skiing, sport, dancing or learning self-defence with family and friends.

- Try creative pastimes such as painting, playing music, gardening, creative writing.
- Socialise with people who are supportive and energising.
- Remember the birthdays of family members and friends— pre-buy cards and gifts.
- Own a pet.
- If watching TV, choose good-quality documentaries and series or entertaining DVDs rather than mind-numbing reality shows and avoid the advertising.
- Turn off the TV and read a book or have an early night.
- Plan ahead for long weekends, holidays, sabbaticals and long-service leave.
- Plan career breaks and holidays for self-reflection.
- Seek peer support and mentoring. Debrief regularly, especially after experiencing death, trauma, grief or suffering among patients or family and friends.
- Acknowledge colleagues' work and value personal work.
- Have an annual health check.

DEAL WITH UNREALISTIC EXPECTATIONS

- Aim for a sustainable workload. Plan breaks after times of excessive workload.
- Book in the occasional appointment with yourself and take some time out to think.
- Maintain feelings of choice and control over workload by taking time to make and implement decisions.
- Write down all the negative expectations of others and negative experiences on a piece of paper and then tear it up and throw it away.
- Recognise personal achievements and give rewards.
- Develop respectful relationships and a sense of community.
- Discover meaning in work and understand what a difference doctors can make to people's lives.

- Remain flexible in career paths.
- Commit to one realistic goal rather than many but always have a challenging goal ahead.
- Do one task at a time and accept uncompleted tasks.
- Say no without feeling guilty and without apologising.
- Plan tasks around commitments in the weeks ahead.
- Prepare for the next day the evening before, then have an early night and get up earlier than usual the next morning to do some exercise.

LEVERAGE TIME

- Basic time management skills include planning ahead, prioritising urgent and non-urgent matters, scheduling of time including lunch and morning and afternoon tea breaks, avoiding unnecessary interruptions and distractions.
- Eliminate time wasting by being proactive about organising time, being selective about which people to meet, when to answer the phone and when to respond to emails. It can help to identify activities that waste time like double handling of mail and emails, reading junk mail and attending non-essential meetings.
- If typing is not a strength, invest in a typing tutor program for the computer or attend a typing course, pay someone else to do the typing or use voice recognition software or a writing plate for the computer.
- Any committee or practice meeting should have a purpose and clear expected outcomes. The meeting agenda should be distributed well before the meeting, and should list the people to attend, state the expected time of commencement and duration, and include well-prepared background papers. Any meeting should result in agreed outcomes with documented minutes and resolutions. At the end of every meeting all participants should feel as if their views and opinions are valued. If this is not the case, it may be necessary to reconsider involvement in the committee or meeting.

- Consider shopping and ordering office supplies, medical equipment and personal items in bulk to save time. Waiting in shopping queues is not a good use of anyone's time. Try to delegate these tasks where possible.

DELEGATE EFFECTIVELY

- The most effective way of leveraging time is by delegation. Paying other people can save money and make money. It may be wise to seek expert advice on hiring staff and employ a practice nurse who can competently triage telephone calls, run chronic disease management programs and provide services such as wound care and immunisations.
- Engage competent and reliable childcare. Pool childcare arrangements with other doctors who are likely to have similar work pressures.
- Delegate home and office cleaning and gardening. However, if gardening or home maintenance is enjoyable, make time for it. Vegetable gardening can be very satisfying.
- A short course in business management is not enough to prepare a doctor for the challenges of running a medical practice. It is usually better to delegate the appropriate aspects of the business to a practice manager, accountant, bank manager and solicitor. Trained experienced staff can save a lot of time, worry and money.
- Write to the president of the relevant medical organisation about any concerns surrounding patient care and professional issues. The subscriptions paid to medical organisations support their ability to advocate on behalf of doctors for positive changes for patient care and professional issues.

BREAK UNHELPFUL HABITS

- Overanalysis is not helpful. Take time out and regain a sense of humour. After a bad day try to use constructive self-talk and mental diversion and avoid rumination.
- Stop trying to please everyone.

- Vent steam with exercise.
- Recognise self-worth; most other people assume doctors know they do a great job.
- Stop taking things so seriously. Have some fun.
- Accept human limitations, the natural course of events and personal vulnerability.
- Stop whinging! Worrying without gaining insight does not change a thing. It wastes precious time.
- Focus on positives, see the temporary nature of many problems and accept the influence of external factors.
- Say no, slow down and keep life simple.
- Don't worry about the 'if onlys' or 'what ifs' in life. Deal with problems as they arise rather than worrying about what might happen in the future or what mistakes may have been made in the past.

PLAN POST GRADUATE TRAINING

- Attend quality continuing professional development activities.
- Access online education and training at a convenient time.

CHALLENGING NEGATIVE THINKING AND BELIEFS

I am not my thoughts.

The Yoga Sutras of Patanjali (2nd century BCE)

If we think negatively we tend to feel negative. We live in an often unhappy world in a time which has been referred to as the age of anxiety, depression and insanity. Being constantly exposed to this negative view can be destructive. As a result, many negative thoughts are stored in our subconscious minds or based on irrational inner beliefs that have been instilled during childhood.

Some examples of unhelpful beliefs include:
- I need other people's approval to make me happy.
- Unless I am a useful productive creative person my life has no meaning.
- I should be happy all the time.
- I should always have complete control over my feelings.
- I should try to impress other people if they are to like me.
- It is weak to feel anxious.
- I must be good at everything in order to feel worthwhile.
- I should never make mistakes and I should always be right.
- I should be humble at all costs.

If we wish to live a more fulfilling relaxed life, we need to adapt our thinking accordingly. Whatever our circumstances, it is unhelpful to let our minds dwell on the same negative thoughts in the same dysfunctional patterns, over and over again. It can help to step back and consider subconscious beliefs that generate unhelpful or negative self-talk. As a start, try to practise prefacing self-talk with words like, 'I will try', 'I would prefer', rather than 'I should', 'I always' and 'I must'.

Here are some examples of common negative thinking patterns.

Black and white thinking supposes that things are either awful or perfect. For example, we may focus on one career as a goal, discounting all other options and predisposing ourselves to feeling like a failure if our 'only' choice happens not to eventuate. The common belief that 'good things happen to good people' and 'bad things happen to bad people' (perpetuated in many cartoon shows and fairy tales) sets people up to think that something must be wrong with them when things go badly. It can be more helpful to think about shades of grey and to try to become aware of the feelings and thoughts in between the extremes.

Common negative over-generalisations include thoughts such as 'Things always go wrong', 'Everyone at work is against me', 'No one understands how I feel'. The evidence for these unhelpful thoughts needs to be challenged. It may help simply to be a little kinder to ourselves with thoughts such as: 'I had a bad day, but tomorrow will be better', 'Work has been stressful for everyone recently but I'll try not to take things so personally' or 'Talking about how I feel to like-minded colleagues will help me feel better'.

Mind-reading involves making assumptions about what someone else thinks of us or believes about us. The evidence for such assumptions needs to be questioned; for example, 'How do you know this?', 'How can you be sure?', 'Might your colleague have something else on their mind?'.

Making mountains out of molehills is a catastrophic way of thinking. For example, 'It will be awful/terrible/horrible', 'I can't stand it any more'. A more helpful approach may be to come up with another way of thinking like: 'Yes, it will be difficult, but I have got through such things before and I will try to do my best'.

CHALLENGING NEGATIVE THINKING

Here are some helpful questions that challenge negative thinking.

- What is the evidence for this way of thinking about the problem?
- What is the argument against this way of thinking?
- Is there another explanation for what you are feeling or what is happening?
- Is there a fresh way of looking at this?
- What is the worst that could happen in this situation?
- Could you get through the worst scenario?
- What is the best that could happen out of this?
- What is the most realistic way things could work out?
- What is the effect of believing your negative thoughts?
- Are these thoughts helpful?
- What would happen if you changed your thinking?
- What would you advise a colleague if they were facing the same situation?
- How have you coped in the past in similar situations?

COMMUNICATING WITH OTHERS
ABOUT PROBLEMS

Better communication is the key to better personal relationships and resolving conflicts. On the downside, if we have problems with communication, we are more likely to feel isolated. If we are isolated, we are more likely to feel depressed.

active listening

As a first step to improving communication, try 'active' listening in your next conversation with a friend or family member. Here are some of the features of active listening:

- Choose the right time to discuss the issue.
- Try to understand what the person is really trying to say by fully listening first.
- Restate what you have heard from the other person in your own words, beginning with something like this: 'Let's see if I understand what you're saying . . .'.
- Try to be neutral and non-judgmental in your answer and your body language.

CONFLICT RESOLUTION

Rather than avoiding conflict, try to see it as an opportunity to build a stronger relationship. Try to work out whether the conflict has arisen as a result of poor communication or personal differences.

TIPS FOR CONFLICT RESOLUTION

Here are some tips for dealing with your next conflict with a colleague, friend or family member.

- Try to identify what's really behind the problem—what are the intentions behind the conflict and what is the other person really trying to say?

☞

- If you feel under personal attack, take responsibility for your own feelings by using 'I' statements like 'I feel hurt . . .', 'I feel distressed . . .', rather than 'You make me . . .'. Refer to the issue at hand rather than allowing a personal attack.

Together list all the possible solutions to a conflict or problem and then weigh up the advantages and disadvantages of each solution objectively. Choose the best solution together—if it does not work, try negotiating again.

RELAXATION EXERCISES

Try to take time for regular relaxation. Here are some common relaxation exercises that might be beneficial to practise everyday.

Relaxing

Mindfulness

Mindfulness is a relaxed state of mind. Try to watch your thoughts as an observer. Don't try to stop stressful thoughts but allow them to flow through your mind and observe them from a distance. Sometimes the statement 'just relax' can make things worse because your active mind finds it difficult to stop thinking and worrying. Instead, accept your active mind and step aside from your thoughts. Try to get some distance from your thoughts by visualising placing your thoughts in boxes on conveyor belts or imagining your thoughts floating through the sky on clouds. Let your thoughts just flow through your mind.

Muscle relaxation

Lie down on your back or sit in a comfortable chair. Become aware of the muscle groups in your body: your hands, arms, shoulders, jaw, face and nose, stomach and legs and feet. Tense your muscle groups for a few seconds and then let them go as follows.

Hands: Make a fist with each hand and let go and relax.

Arms: Stretch your arms out in front of you, raise them high up over your head and stretch higher. Let your arms drop back to your side and feel them go floppy.

Shoulders: Pull your shoulders up to your ears. Hold in tight and then relax.

Jaw: Clench your teeth together really hard. Then let your jaw hang loose.

Face and nose: Make lots of wrinkles on your forehead, and crinkle up your nose, then let your face go smooth.

Stomach: Pull your abdominal muscles in. Try to make them touch your spine. Make yourself as skinny as you can, then release your abdomen.

Legs and feet: Push your feet and toes down on the floor. Let your feet and toes go loose and floppy.

Take time to let each muscle group lose the tension and relax.

Visualisation

Visualisation of past pleasant experiences is a powerful way to instant relaxation. Think of one of your favourite places, like the beach, a bushwalk, a garden or a park. Imagine the smells, sounds, touch and scenery. Bring yourself back to the state of your mind when you were last at this place. Try to feel a wonderful state of quietness and peace in this place. Feel a sense of contentment. Take a deep breath in and out.

On a day off, try practising silence by immersing yourself in nature and just listening rather than talking. Next time you are feeling stressed (for example, while driving in peak hour or sitting at your computer) bring yourself back to this place.

Breathing

Sit comfortably in a quiet room. Count your normal breathing rate for 60 seconds. Then breathe in on the slow count of three (one… two … three …) and out for the slow count of three, for a full minute. Try counting your normal breathing rate over 60 seconds again and compare it to what it was before the exercise. The breathing rate often slows down, which in turn helps the heart slow down and this helps relaxation.

DON'T ALWAYS DELAY GRATIFICATION—
SEEK PLEASURE IN SIMPLE THINGS

Doctors become very practised at putting life on hold temporarily while studying or working. Self-discipline and willpower are important, but when we continually defer happiness and ignore the signs of fatigue and stress, it's easy to become dissociated and tired of life. When we do have free time it can be difficult to cope with idleness. If this is the case we may find it helpful to rediscover what relaxes us. Many doctors are talented musicians, artists, writers and sportspeople. It is important to maintain those more creative sides of our beings.

Seeking simple pleasures

Identify things in your day which give you pleasure—simple, enjoyable things like playing sport, reading, breathing clean air, feeling the sun on your skin, talking to a friend, laughing, singing, taking a bath, listening to music, walking the dog, gardening, playing golf, going to the gym, swimming, cooking healthy food, riding a bike, learning another language, dancing, knitting, smelling flowers, going to the theatre, reading a newspaper, taking photos, writing, reading poetry, watching a sunset, visiting an art gallery, smelling a favourite perfume, tasting chocolate or fresh fruit, growing something from seed or fresh herbs on your windowsill.

• What are the simple things *you* enjoy?
• Write them down and make time to do more of them every day.

SLEEPING WELL

Problems with lack of sleep commonly precede depression and make feelings of fatigue and irritability worse. Avoid daytime or evening naps, time in bed ruminating without sleeping, inactivity during the day (but don't exercise close to bedtime), work or stressful phone calls or emails before bedtime, rethinking about today or tomorrow's stressful events and drinks containing caffeine or alcohol.

Sleeping well

To break the sleep/wake/insomnia cycle, only go to bed when sleepy. If you lie in bed awake for more than 30 minutes at any time of the night or early morning, get up and do something soothing—do this every time it happens throughout the night if necessary. Try to set yourself a routine time for getting up in the morning, no matter what time you went to bed or how tired you are. Stop lying there and worrying while in bed. Stop worrying that you cannot sleep. Try relaxation exercises and more physical exercise throughout the day instead. It takes discipline but it works.

Coping strategies

Here are some coping strategies to try.

- Actively think about the positive aspects of your life, including your relationships or interactions with others and the simple pleasures of life.
- Do something to alter the situation causing you stress; fix the problem or increase your feelings of control. For example, confront the person causing stress, or develop practice policies to deal with difficult situations or complete that task that you have been putting off for weeks which makes you feel guilty every time you think of it.
- Alternatively, identify the triggers to stress and refrain from doing anything that may make the stress worse. For example, delay a decision or decide not to react.
- Seek more information to determine the extent of a problem, the facts surrounding the problem and what can be done about it.
- Realise you are placing too much emphasis on something that is causing you to feel stressed. Try to devalue the importance of the event and focus on potentially positive outcomes.
- Challenge negative thinking by identifying negative self-talk and use of generalisations ('I'll never…', 'I can't do anything right…', 'Nobody will ever want me', 'I'm hopeless'). Identify the things you do right and the things you do well.
- Seek social support or professional assistance.

- Try mental diversion from your problem or do something you find relaxing.
- Undertake regular physical activity to keep your mind and body healthy.

Active acceptance is about recognising things as they are and then choosing the course of action we deem appropriate and worthy of ourselves. It is about recognising that at every moment in our life we have a choice—to be afraid and to act courageously—to feel jealousy and act benevolently—to want approval and to act autonomously—to be human because we accept our humanity.[1]

Tal Ben-Shahar, contemporary author and lecturer

PHYSICAL HEALTH

It seems obvious to aim for wellbeing rather than just the absence of disease. But few of us take our own advice. Many doctors are over their healthy weight, do not exercise and fail to attend to preventive health care. Here is a six-step approach to staying physically healthy.

STEP I
HAVE AN ANNUAL PREVENTIVE HEALTH CHECK

As we know, we don't have to feel sick to be sick. Table I on p.56 includes a list of recommended screening tests. If we are inactive, over our healthy weight, smoke, drink alcohol regularly or have a family history of an illness, we may require earlier screening more often.

We recommend all doctors, particularly those of us over the age of 45, have an annual preventive health check to ensure we receive annual screening for common physical and mental health problems. It is also important that we encourage family members to have routine screening at the ages listed in Table I, with their own doctor.[2]

---

1   Tal Ben-Shahar, www.happinessanditscauses.com.au
2   Rowe, L. and Kidd, M.R. (2007), *Save Your Life and the Lives of those You Love: Your GPs' 6 Step Guide for Staying Healthy Longer*, Sydney: Allen and Unwin.

STEP 2
KNOW YOUR FAMILY HISTORY

Many disorders run in families and the age of diagnosis in a family member may be a key to the age we require screening for disorders such as:

- Cancers, including cancers of the gastrointestinal tract, breast, colon, lung, ovary or prostate
- Cardiovascular disorders such as hypertension, heart disease, hypercholesterolaemia or stroke
- Type 2 diabetes
- Kidney failure
- Mental health problems such as depression or alcohol abuse

STEP 3
AIM FOR PERMANENT HEALTHY WEIGHT LOSS

The shelves of bookshops are stacked with weight-loss books recommending fad diets that don't work and, what's worse, leave us feeling hungry, flatulent or tired. Around 60% of people are overweight and at risk of preventable serious illnesses such as heart disease, stroke, diabetes and cancers. The secret of healthy weight loss is simple but not very popular—healthy eating and physical activity. Weight loss is good old-fashioned hard work. We recommend a back-to-basics approach to healthy weight loss.

Steps to healthy weight loss

Choose colourful low-kilojoule foods

It takes 37 000 kilojoules to lose 1 kg of fat and if you take a look at the kilojoule contents of most foods, you will realise it takes a lot of willpower to lose weight permanently. You will lose weight if you expend more kilojoules during exercise than you eat. ☞

☞ Plan your daily food diary to include:
- At least two serves of fruit and five serves of vegetables, including green leafy vegetables and colourful varieties
- Wholegrain cereal and bread
- Fish
- Two to three serves of low-fat milk, or plain yoghurt for calcium
- Healthy drinks such as water or green tea. Aim to drink at least 2 litres of water each day.

Reduce the size of your meals and your intake of salt, junk foods, saturated fat (less meat and full-cream diary products) and trans fats (no commercial biscuits, cakes or muffins) to reduce your risk of heart disease.

Many so-called *health foods* are not healthy, especially those which are high in fat, sugar and kilojoules. For example, a muffin and a small bottle of orange juice for morning tea contain about 2500 kilojoules. A piece of fruit and a glass of water contain about 300 kilojoules. If you keep an eye on the energy content of foods you can cut out many unnecessary kilojoules without making your life a misery.

Reduce your emotional eating and drinking

Try not to feed your emotional appetite with food or drinking alcohol or drinks high in sugar. When you feel bored, irritable, angry or stressed try to express these emotions in more constructive ways such as talking to a friend or exercising. Many people who are obese are also depressed and cannot find the motivation to lose weight. If someone is depressed it is usually best to treat the depression first. When you do eat, slow down and savour your meals.

Weigh yourself regularly

Despite popular opinion we believe it is a good idea to weigh yourself and to measure your waist circumference regularly. Reward yourself with something other than food if you lose weight or centimetres. If you find it difficult to shift weight, don't be discouraged. You may like to try low-calorie meal substitute drinks available from your local pharmacy or discuss medication with your own doctor. For some people who are morbidly obese with a body mass index over 40, laparoscopic banding may be the most effective option.

STEP 4
PHYSICAL ACTIVITY IS NOT OPTIONAL

As we all know, regular physical activity has enormous proven benefits:

- It keeps weight down.
- It reduces the risk of Type 2 diabetes.
- It keeps blood pressure down.
- It raises HDL and lowers LDL and triglycerides.
- It reduces stress and mental illness.
- It prevents osteoporosis.
- It delays the onset of dementia.
- It reduces the risk of cancer and improves outcomes after cancer diagnosis, particularly bowel cancer.

A minimum of 30 minutes moderate exercise is recommended at least five times each week. During moderate exercise, the heart rate will be at least 60–70% of our maximum heart rate (220 minus your age) for 30 minutes a day. If we wish to lose weight, we need to exercise more vigorously for longer.

STEP 5
REDUCE YOUR RISKY BEHAVIOURS

Some very damaging habits like overeating, smoking, excess alcohol and other drug use are often used as quick fixes for stress. They can be very addictive.

Bad habits

The following simple questions may help you consider your resistance to reducing any bad habits.

- How does your lifestyle affect your body, mood and life?
- What concerns you at the moment?
- What did you learn from previous attempts to change your lifestyle?
- How can you do things differently?
- What would have to happen for your motivation to increase?

Nicotine is highly addictive and nicotine withdrawal sometimes requires combination treatment with nicotine replacement therapy and medications like bupropion or varenicline.

We believe that the benefits of alcohol are often overemphasised by the alcohol industry. Low-risk drinking is usually defined as no more than two standard drinks a day, with at least two alcohol-free days per week. The use of alcohol as a coping strategy is a very unhelpful habit.

STEP 6
RESPOND IMMEDIATELY TO THE RED ALERTS

All doctors know that some symptoms should never be ignored. We know the signs of cardiovascular disease, cerebrovascular disease and cancer. Yet many of our colleagues have ignored these signs and failed to seek timely assistance. Like the rest of the population, if we have central chest pain lasting for more than a few minutes, or temporary or permanent weakness of face or limb, we need to call an ambulance immediately. We must see our own doctor as soon as possible for unexplained loss of weight, unexplained fatigue or prolonged pain, new lesions or abnormal bleeding or discharge. As we know well, early detection of preventable disorders can prevent years of suffering.

> We are doctors. We know the importance of physical, mental, spiritual and emotional health for our patients. Yet we often neglect our own health and wellbeing. This can have a detrimental effect not only on ourselves but also on our families and our patients.

CHAPTER 5

OUR RELATIONSHIP WITH OUR OWN DOCTOR

A physician who treats himself has a fool for a patient.

Sir William Osler (1849–1919), Physician

WHY IS IT THAT SO MANY DOCTORS DON'T HAVE THEIR OWN DOCTOR?

Medical culture seems to foster inappropriate help-seeking behaviour, denial, and self-assessment, investigation, treatment and referral. 'I've got too much work to do', 'I know myself better than any doctor' we might say.

But not only is treating ourselves unwise, in many countries it is an offence for doctors to self-prescribe drugs.

Some of us find it a challenge accessing health care. Many of us have difficulty relinquishing control or fear being judged as weak and not coping by colleagues. Some of us accept low levels of wellbeing, chronic stress and fatigue as being a normal state. We may be particularly concerned about presenting to a colleague if we have a mental health problem. Many of us are reluctant to take sick leave as it places burdens on colleagues and is difficult to do in any self-employed business.

TREATING OTHER DOCTORS

It is an honour to treat another doctor because we tend to consider our choice carefully. Here are some tips for dealing with doctors as patients:

- Avoid treating doctor patients as VIPs. As with any patient, ask them what their self-diagnostic ideas are. 'What do you think is wrong?' is a reasonable question but be objective and feel free to disagree with their conclusion.

- Don't assume the doctor as a patient understands all aspects of their medical condition. Always explain options fully. A doctor as a patient will often present with serious and complex medical issues because often they have tried self-investigation and treatment first or delayed seeking care. However, it is a common pitfall to spend more time with a doctor patient than is necessary.

PHYSICAL HEALTH CARE

Over the past century increases in life expectancy were achieved largely by advances in sanitation, immunisation and antibiotics. Most of the more recent gains related to the availability of expensive health technology are now being undermined by the impact of the global rise in obesity, lack of physical activity and use of tobacco and abuse of alcohol. Doctors tend to have better levels of physical health than the general population because we are unlikely to smoke and we are more likely to present for the diagnosis and management of hypertension. However, it is not hard to beat the rest of the population when it comes to health statistics. One in two men and one in three women over the age of 40 years will develop heart disease. Doctors, like everyone else in the community, can do more about preventive health care.

There are many helpful resources to assist doctors provide evidence-based lifestyle advice and screening tests.[1]

Table 1 outlines recommended preventive health screening tests for all healthy adults based on international guidelines. If we are above our healthy weight, have an unhealthy lifestyle related to poor nutrition, an inactive lifestyle, smoke or drink an excessive amount of alcohol; if we have a past history or family history of particular diseases; or if we belong to certain ethnic backgrounds, some of these tests are recommended at much younger ages and at more frequent intervals.

1   The Royal Australian College of General Practitioners (2009), *Guidelines for Preventive Activities in General Practice*, 7th edn, Melbourne: RACGP; The Royal Australian College of General Practitioners (2006), *Putting Prevention into Practice: Guidelines for the Implementation of Prevention in the General Practice Setting*, 2nd edn, Melbourne: RACGP; The Royal Australian College of General Practitioners (2004), *SNAP Guide: A Population Health Guide*, Melbourne: RACGP; Zwar, N. (2008), 'Smoking cessation—what works?', *Australian Family Physician*, 37: 10–14; Lee, K.L. (2008), 'Alcohol intervention—what works?', *Australian Family Physician*, 37: 16–19; Egger, G. (2008), 'Helping patients lose weight—what works?', *Australian Family Physician*, 37: 20–23; Smith, B.J. *et al.* (2008), 'Encouraging physical activity—five steps for GPs', *Australian Family Physician*, 37: 24–28.

Table I Recommended preventive health screening for healthy adults

Age	Assessment	Frequency
From age 13 years	Skin checks for those with high risk skin	Annually
From age 18 years—all the above and …	Waist measurement for people who appear to be overweight	Every 2 years
	Body Mass Index for people who appear to be overweight	Every 2 years
	Blood pressure	Every 2 years
	Chlamydia test for men and women at risk	Annually
	Mental health (including risk for depression and suicide)	Opportunistically
From age 20 years— all the above and …	Pap smear in sexually active women	Every 2 years until age 70 years
From age 40 years— all the above and …	Diabetes risk factor assessment and preventive advice	Every 3 years
From age 45 years—all the above and …	Cardiovascular risk factor assessment and preventive advice	Every 2 years
	Fasting blood lipids	Every 5 years
	Osteoporosis risk factor assessment and preventive advice in women	Annually.
From age 50 years—all the above and …	Blood pressure more frequently	Every 12 months
	Urinary protein (tested by dipstick)	Every 5 years
	Faecal occult blood	Every 2 years
	Prostate risk assessment in men. Risks/benefits of prostate screening may be discussed with your doctor	Opportunistically
	Osteoporosis risk factor assessment and preventive advice in men	Annually
	Mammogram in women	Every 2 years, optional for ages 40 to 49 and over 70
	Vision test	Every 5 years
From age 65 years—all the above and …	Bone mineral densitometry for osteoporosis in women	Every 2 years
	Vision and hearing tests	Annually

Adapted from The Royal Australian College of General Practitioners (2009), *Guidelines for Preventive Activities in General Practice*, 7th edn, Melbourne: RACGP.

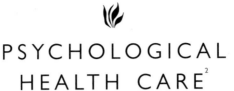

PSYCHOLOGICAL
HEALTH CARE[2]

Everything can be taken away from a man but one thing; the last of the human freedoms—to choose one's attitude in any given circumstances, to choose one's way.

Viktor Frankl (1905–1997), neurologist, psychiatrist and Holocaust survivor

It should not be surprising that we suffer from the same mental illnesses as the general population. Like the rest of the community, we fear the stigma of admitting to symptoms of mental illness and often receive late or suboptimal treatment, which can result in a poor prognosis or relapse. Many of us do not recognise mental illness in ourselves, despite our knowledge of the symptoms and signs. We might say: 'I'm just run down', or 'It couldn't happen to me'.

In addition, many members of our families, friends and work colleagues fail to recognise or support us when we have a mental illness because they only consider us in our caring role. One of the most common signs of mental illness can be failure to cope with work or study because of the problems associated with concentration. We tend to continue to function at work through any illness and have very low levels of sick leave. We also have the ability to mask symptoms. In reality, those of us who fail to cope with work demands are often viewed very critically by other colleagues for 'letting the team down'.

Many psychiatrists routinely seek supervision and debriefing to work through any vicarious effects of consulting clients with mental health problems. However, doctors working in all other specialties are also affected by patient suffering, but are less aware of the need to debrief regularly.

2   This section is based on: Treatment Protocol Project (2004), *Management of Mental Disorder*, 4th edn, Sydney: World Health Organization, Collaborating Centre for Evidence in Mental Health Policy.

In many countries doctors are mandated to report colleagues who are mentally impaired to the local medical practitioners' board or government organisation. Ideally a doctor who is mentally impaired will be detected in a routine annual preventive health check with their own doctor and their medical problems will be managed early and appropriately with the caring support of their own doctor.

For these reasons, routine screening for mental illness should occur during annual routine preventive health assessments by another doctor. Another reason why it is important to consult another doctor for symptoms of depression is to rule out any physical cause of the illness and to have another clinician assess the illness objectively.

Here is a reminder of the features of a mental health history:

- What is the nature of this person's presenting problem?
- What are the specific symptoms?
- What events led to this presentation?
- Are there any symptoms or signs of underlying physical illness which may have predisposed this person to mental illness such as an endocrine disorder, infection, neurological disorder, cardiovascular disease, collagen disorder, malignancy or metabolic disorder?
- What is this person's suicide risk?
- What is this person's past history? What past and current medications has this person been taking, including drugs that may be associated with depressive symptoms such as analgesics, anti-inflammatory agents, antihypertensives, antineoplastics, neurological agents and steroids or hormones?
- What is this person's developmental history as a child and adolescent and young adult?
- What is this person's education and work history?
- What is this person's marital and family history?
- How are this person's relationships with their children and significant others?

DEPRESSION

Major depression is characterised by a cluster of symptoms, which vary from person to person. Symptoms include feeling sad or irritable, sleep disturbance, loss of interest in usual activities, feeling worthless or guilty, changes in appetite or weight, loss of sexual interest, physical aches and pains, impaired thinking or concentration and thoughts of death. Five or more of these symptoms need to be present for two or more weeks for a formal diagnosis of major depression to be made.

Dysthymia is a chronic mood disturbance present on most days over a span of at least two years. The symptoms are not as severe as those for major depression but may be just as damaging.

About 20% of people will experience a depressive illness at some time in their lives. Postnatal depression in women doctors is more likely in association with relationship difficulties, poor social supports and stressful life events.

Optimal management includes thorough psychiatric and medical assessment, including suicide assessment. The goal of therapy with psychological and drug treatment is to eliminate the depressed mood. A good outcome is more likely with education and support of the individual and their family. We should never ever self-prescribe drug treatment for our own depression.

Cognitive behavioural therapy and interpersonal therapy are appropriate psychological treatments for depression. Selective Serotonin Reuptake Inhibitors (SSRIs) are preferred drugs in most people for the treatment of depression including postnatal depression because of the lower side-effect profile and safety in overdose.

SSRIs are usually taken in the morning with food as they often disturb sleep at night. There can be a delay of one to two weeks before any benefit is experienced and the full effect may not be apparent for four to eight weeks.

Side effects of SSRIs may include increased appetite, weight gain, nausea, constipation, postural dizziness, drowsiness, dry mouth, sexual dysfunction and increased sensitivity to sun exposure. To increase compliance, these side effects may be managed appropriately by simple techniques such as increasing exercise, adjusting diet, increasing fluid intake and dividing doses. Serotonin syndrome and suicidality are rare side effects of SSRIs.

To prevent the high likelihood of a relapse or recurrence of depression, a number of psychological strategies are used including structured problem solving, sleep hygiene techniques, increasing activity and exercise, encouraging healthy eating behaviours, relaxation training and assertiveness and communication training. Long-term maintenance antidepressant medication may be recommended to prevent relapse in people at risk, including those with chronic exposure to stress.

Common warning signs of a relapse of depression include changes in sleep pattern, decreased concentration, withdrawal and isolation, lack of energy, irritability, loss of interest in usual activities and lowered mood.

A checklist for the diagnosis of depression is given in Appendix I.

ANXIETY DISORDERS

Anxiety is a normal reaction. High levels of anxiety may be appropriate for dealing with excessive demands. Moderate levels of anxiety can improve performance and be protective. Anxiety disorders are very prevalent disorders and are characterised by prolonged distress and tension out of all proportion to life stressors and which impair functioning.

People with anxiety may have:

- Persistent excessive or unrealistic worries which interfere with life, work or activities (generalised anxiety disorder)
- Compulsions or obsessions which they can't control including overchecking, fear of germs, overcleaning, overcounting and repeating routine activities and actions (obsessive compulsive disorder)
- Intense excessive worry related to social situations (social anxiety disorder)
- Panic attacks (panic disorder)
- An intensely irrational fear of everyday objects and situations (phobia)

Symptoms of anxiety disorders may include palpitations, difficulty in breathing, gastro-intestinal disorder, muscle tension, sweating, feelings of choking, feeling faint or tremor.

About one in 10 people develop anxiety disorders and women are more likely to be affected.

Effective treatments include cognitive behavioural therapy and antidepressant medication, including SSRIs.

A checklist for the diagnosis of anxiety disorders is given in Appendix I.

EATING DISORDERS

An eating disorder is characterised by obsessive thoughts about food and body weight, which are often hidden from others. Anorexia nervosa, bulimia and compulsive overeating are common eating disorders.

About one in every 50 people, most commonly young women, will develop an eating disorder at some stage of their lives.

A team of health professionals is often enlisted for the treatment of eating disorders including a psychiatrist, dietician, psychologist and mental health nurse. Psychotherapy is essential. There is no evidence to support antidepressants in the treatment of anorexia nervosa, but SSRIs may be considered for co-morbid depression.

BIPOLAR DISORDER

Bipolar disorder is a form of psychotic illness. People with bipolar disorder may experience extreme highs and lows of mood and may behave in an irrational or risky manner. The cycles of highs and lows vary from individual to individual.

Doctors with untreated bipolar disorder may present with difficulty making decisions and concentrating or may become uncharacteristically reckless. Grandiose ideas, inflated self-esteem, increased energy, enhanced libido, impaired judgment and impulsive behaviour along with impaired insight may put a doctor at risk of ruining their reputation and place their patients at serious risk of harm.

About one in 50 people will develop bipolar disorder sometime in their lives.

As with other mental illnesses, it is essential to have a thorough psychiatric, social and general medical assessment including suicide risk assessment.

Mood-stabilising medication such as lithium is used to treat depressive and manic symptoms. An antidepressant may be added to treat depressive symptoms, but must be ceased if there are manic symptoms. Manic symptoms may require a benzodiazepine or an antipsychotic.

To reduce the likelihood of recurrence, a prophylactic mood stabiliser is used. Doctors as patients must be educated about the risk factors and the early signs of relapse and the importance of compliance with medication.

SCHIZOPHRENIA

Schizophrenia is a form of psychotic illness which interferes with a person's ability to think, feel and behave. The DSM IV criteria for schizophrenia include two or more of the following, each present for a significant portion of time during a one-month period:

- Delusions
- Hallucinations
- Disorganised speech (e.g. incoherence)
- Grossly disorganised or catatonic behaviour
- Negative symptoms (i.e. affective flattening)

About one in 100 people develop schizophrenia at some time in their lives, mostly in their late teens and early 20s.

Early treatment of schizophrenia usually within one week of the onset of symptoms is associated with a much better prognosis. As with all mental illnesses, most people who receive optimal treatment lead happy and fulfilling lives. However, late treatment is often associated with poor prognosis and lifelong disability. The importance of early treatment with low-dose antipsychotic medication and a comprehensive management plan cannot be overestimated.

SUBSTANCE-USE DISORDERS

A substance-use disorder is generally characterised by a strong desire to take alcohol or drugs or prescribed medication, difficulty in controlling use or harmful physical and psychological consequences which may include reduced work performance, negative impact on relationships, depression secondary to heavy consumption or physical illness including liver damage.

Dependence is a physical and psychological syndrome resulting from the repetitive use of a psychoactive substance. A person who is dependent has a strong desire to take the substance and difficulty controlling the use of the substance. Symptoms of withdrawal include anxiety, depression and sleep disturbance. The use of the substance relieves the withdrawal symptoms. Over time, higher doses are required to achieve the same effect and a tolerance to the drug is evident. The substance use continues despite evidence of harmful consequences.

The use of substances must be assessed within the context of the individual's life and their readiness for change. A psychiatric history is important to identify possible co-morbidity including depression, anxiety, psychosis, post-traumatic stress disorder, eating disorders and bipolar disorder. The severity of dependence, the physical health consequences and any risk-taking behaviour associated with substance use must be explored. The treatment and management plan must be adjusted according to the history and the motivation of the individual. While self-management and monitoring are to be encouraged, it is essential that a doctor with a substance-use disorder is monitored and reviewed regularly by another doctor.

COGNITIVE DECLINE

Cognitive decline is another cause of mental impairment. Many doctors postpone retirement because of the pressure of medical workforce shortages. There are many doctors who continue to work over the age of 70 or even 80 years. Serious cognitive decline in doctors is associated with very serious implications for public safety. It can be very difficult to approach this subject with a colleague. Often the best course of action is to say quietly: 'I am worried about you. Can I help or support you?'. Ageing doctors should not be discriminated against for their commitment and dedication to their patients. Many ageing doctors continue to work effectively and contribute enormously to the health and wellbeing of the people in their local communities.

HOW TO RESPOND TO A COLLEAGUE WHO IS IMPAIRED

In many countries medical practitioners are required to report an impaired colleague to the relevant medical board or similar organisation. This action usually results in formal peer review and appropriate intervention.

This can be a harrowing outcome for a doctor after a dedicated career. All of us have a responsibility to respond early and appropriately under these circumstances in the interests of patient safety. Knowing when to retire is an important decision and a critical challenge for some. Many of us choose to retire before our health affects our clinical practice. For example, some surgeons choose to retire at the age of 65 years, despite their skill and experience. Some of us who have experienced mental illness choose to have well-planned career breaks and attend our own doctor regularly for objective review of our situation.

Whatever our circumstances, we must plan for career breaks and eventual retirement from practice as carefully as we plan each other aspect of our medical careers. We must ensure we take heed of our colleagues' concerns.

Each of us needs our own doctor, someone we trust who can provide us with medical care, support and advice and assist us to maintain optimal physical and mental health and wellbeing.

If you are having trouble finding a suitable doctor, ask your colleagues who they see, or contact your local medical association or Doctor's Health Organisation for advice.

CHAPTER 6

OUR RELATIONSHIPS WITH OUR FAMILIES AND FRIENDS

More than anything else, the way we deal with loss shapes our capacity to be fully alive. The way we protect ourselves from loss may be the way in which we distance ourselves from life.

Dr Rachel Remen, contemporary doctor and author[1]

Our families can be a major influence on our choice of medicine as a career. Strong, continuing, nurturing relationships with family and friends are the most important sources of our support throughout our careers. But good relationships don't just happen— they require time for communication, respect and love.

Sadly, these relationships are the ones we are most likely to neglect in the face of excessive workloads. Many of us are dedicated to medicine, but detached from our own emotions and the emotions of our family members and friends. This is unfortunate as talking about stress with family and friends can be one of the most effective strategies for dealing with it.

In recent years the Myers-Briggs Type Indicator® (MBTI®) has become a widely used tool to assess and categorise people's behavioural preferences. MBTI® results identify valuable differences between normal healthy people, differences that can be the source of

1 Remen, R. (1997), *The Little Book of Kitchen Table Wisdom*, New York: Riverhead Trade.

much misunderstanding and miscommunication. This information is useful for us both in terms of understanding our own style and the interactions we have with others.

The assessment reports on the extent to which:

- our energy is focused on the outer world of people and activity (extraverted) OR our inner world of ideas and experiences (introverted)
- we focus on the logical consequences of an action OR what is important to us and to others when making decisions
- we prefer an orderly OR flexible life
- we focus on the big picture and connections OR the details and what is real and tangible.

Our relationships with others are affected by the interaction between different preferences. For example, an extraverted person who enjoys being with people may have to adapt to their introverted partner's need for solitude. A person who needs the security and certainty of making decisions may have to learn to leave some options open for a partner who prefers to be flexible and open to new opportunities. People who base their decisions on logic alone may have to understand that their relationship with a partner who bases decisions on emotion requires some flexibility and that this is more important than being right all the time.

Once people are aware of their behavioural preferences they can work on being more balanced and develop their less preferred ways of interacting. Personality traits are more enduring and take time and effort to change. Some of the negative personalities and behaviours which may lead to dysfunctional relationships include:

- Constant negative thinking and talking, where the underlying problem may be a sense of inferiority, low self-esteem, unhappiness, boredom or depression
- Hard-to-please perfectionist tendencies
- Arrogance, but with associated hypersensitivity to criticism which may be related to limited life experiences and the inability to self-reflect
- Bossy and overcontrolling behaviours which are often related to underlying anxiety

- Compassion fatigue and low levels of empathy due to burnout
- Excessive worrying related to fears and anxiety
- Avoidance of conflict perhaps because of negative experiences of anger as a child
- Passive aggressive behaviours where there is quiet protest through inaction or being late or resistance against cooperating and being controlled.

It is worth thinking about the way different traits and behaviours can contribute to challenges in relationships with family members. We can respond more constructively to difficult interactions with others if we understand the underlying reason for a behaviour.

LIFE PARTNERSHIPS

Although doctors tend to experience low rates of divorce, we tend to tolerate high levels of marital and sexual relationship problems and conflict. Long working hours and excessive demands intrude into the family lives of many doctors.

The essentials of all great partnerships include unconditional love, mutual respect and courtesy and the ability to compromise and to share interests and values. Good communication, shared decision making, trust, commitment and intimacy all require time.

On the negative side, here are some patterns in doctors' partnerships which can lead to troubled relationships.[2]

THE DRIVEN DOCTOR

Many of us tend to have personality characteristics such as obsessional traits, feelings of self-doubt and guilt, excessive fear of failure, excessive fear of making a mistake and an exaggerated sense

---

2 Harris, E. (1998), 'The doctor's trouble marriage', *Australian Family Physician*, 27: 999–1004.

of responsibility. These characteristics may be developmental in origin, may be reinforced during training or may be an adaptation to excessive workloads.

A doctor's non-medical partner may seek the status of being a doctor's partner and a sense of personal identity and self-worth through the partnership. As the doctor becomes more immersed in work and detached, their partner may feel more dissatisfied and anxious. As the partnership deteriorates, the doctor may immerse themself further into work. Chronic marital distress may be tolerated by both partners or the pattern may end, more often when the non-medical partner leaves to form another relationship.

THE 'SPECIAL' DOCTOR

In some cases doctors have been perceived by their families to be 'special' as children and have developed an exaggerated sense of self. Other doctors may have experienced emotional neglect as children. These doctors may be driven by an unconscious fear of failure and be deeply offended by any criticism. In response to a challenge, these doctors may become unreasonable or angry and unconsciously inflict insecurities about self-worth onto their partner or children.

Many doctors work hard because of a pervasive need for status and to compete with colleagues. In this situation the doctor's partner may become increasingly critical of the authoritarian attitude of the doctor and chronic conflict and resentment may arise.

THE CAREER PARTNERSHIP

This is a partnership of people with equally demanding careers. Superficially the couple live together peacefully, but there may actually be very little happiness or companionship. Partnership may have been sought for comfort and security rather than for what each partner has in common.

Women doctors are particularly vulnerable to this type of relationship. While some non-medical partners share domestic and parenting roles, most women doctors continue to juggle all responsibilities and may feel guilty at failing to meet their own impossible expectations. This arrangement has the potential to create conflict in a partnership.

Chronically unhappy relationships require time for nurturing. Simply understanding the common patterns of relationship problems may assist many doctors build happy and satisfying relationships.

SEXUAL PROBLEMS

One of the most common but overlooked problems for us in our relationships with our partners are sexual problems related to differences in sexual desire. It is easy to feel out of sync with our partners because of external stresses and heavy workloads. Sexual problems are commonly dismissed as the least of our problems, but they may herald the onset of major relationship issues and medical illness.

The most common causes of relationship difficulties associated with sexual problems include:

- Inability to communicate about sex and to seek to understand each others' needs
- Lack of privacy, wakeful children, after-hours calls
- Preoccupation with the excessive demands of our work
- Fatigue or stress related to overwork
- Anxiety about sexual performance
- Not making time for sex.

Lack of emotional wellbeing, communication problems, lack of intimacy, respect and trust and unresolved tensions are all inhibitors of sexual desire. The key is to anticipate that excessive work demands usually create disturbances in sexual desire between partners. We need to communicate about this before this leads to a negative cycle of emotions.

Good communication about sex is the key.[3] It is important to find

3   Bradford, D. and Russell, D. (2006), *Talking with Clients about Sex*, Melbourne: IP Communications Pty Ltd; King, R. (1997), *Good Loving Great Sex*, Sydney: Random House.

out specifically what increases and decreases our partner's sexual desire and to express freely sexual needs in a loving way without pressing or rejecting our partner. Sometimes rest and relaxation and quality time are all that are required to restore sexual desire. At other times more effort will be required to reconnect intimately.

If differences in sexual desire and needs are not communicated sensitively, they can develop into a major source of conflict within a relationship. If this negative cycle has already been established in a relationship, a counsellor or a sex therapist may be able to restore communication channels.

There are many other causes for sexual problems ranging from fatigue to past sexual abuse, medical conditions, drug use and issues related to sexual identity. The gradual onset of sexual dysfunction may also herald a significant medical condition such as diabetes, hyperlipidaemia, hypertension, thyroid disease, hypogonadism, prostatic disease, depression or anxiety. Dyspareunia should not be ignored as it may signal serious illnesses such as endometriosis, pelvic inflammatory disease or ovarian or uterine tumours. Many commonly used medications can also be associated with sexual problems. When sexual problems persist, it is important to see another doctor. Sexual problems may be a sign of medical illness and prolonged sexual problems can also have very negative consequences for our relationships.

Maintaining healthy sexual boundaries is also essential. Relationships with patients are not appropriate.

PARENTING

The children of doctors are assumed to have absent doctor parents or an absent doctor parent and an overinvolved, unhappily married, non-medical parent. As doctors, we are increasingly changing this stereotypical view and demanding more work–life balance to allow us to be effective partners and parents.

Nevertheless many of our children complain about the excessive pressure related to being a member of a medical family. The all too familiar question 'Are you going to be a doctor like your mum/dad?' usually provokes an angry response.

More than any group in the community we see the negative consequences of poor parenting on young people including depression, drug and alcohol use and other major health issues. However, like most of the community, we rarely undertake training for the most important job in the world—parenting. Like all parents in management positions at work, it is easy to adopt an ineffective, overcontrolling approach to parenting. At the other extreme, parents who juggle excessive work demands sometimes take a permissive approach to parenting to avoid conflict and just to keep the peace at home. Sometimes parents swing inconsistently between the two extremes.

What style of parenting protects children and adolescents from harm and promotes resilience?

Research tells us that the most effective style of parenting is warm and respectful, loving, nurturing and flexible, but firm. In this caring approach parents encourage their children to make good choices, negotiate conflict constructively and care strongly about personal values.

Warm and respectful parents listen and reassure, but also make it clear when they disagree and for what reasons. They are high on warmth and reasonably high on control while being sufficiently flexible to take account, within reason, of their child's level of maturity and development.

At the other extreme, *pressure cooker* parents are low on warmth and high on control, frequently interfering in minor issues that, in the overall scheme of things, don't really matter. Pressure cooker parents tend to believe incorrectly that 'mollycoddling' a child will interfere with their growing up into a successful, appropriately independent adult. They create an unnecessary emotional distance, often giving advice before or instead of listening and either squash or inflame conflict. There is also a major focus in this parenting approach on discipline and punishment, generally of the 'do as I say, not as I do' variety.

In response to parenting that is meddlesome, often inconsistent and lacking in warmth and care, children will often withdraw in quiet resentment or display behavioural problems. Fear of loss of control leads the pressure cooker parent to comment incessantly on or interfere continually in relation to their child's friends and future ambitions as well as what their child should eat, drink, wear, study and do with their leisure time. These parents tend to believe that if they lose the small battles on the home front they will lose total control. Unfortunately they often lose a great deal more than control—it is the pressure cooker parent who inadvertently puts their child most at risk of depression. In this environment, the child will find it very difficult to develop a sense of autonomy or gain the important feeling that they have at least some control over their own lives.

The *anything goes* parent, who is generally high on warmth but far too low on control, tends to raise children with poor social skills, insecurity and other similar behavioural traits. Without clear rules and boundaries to test out against, adolescents in particular tend to seek their role models and guidance elsewhere, not always with satisfactory results. Anything goes parents are not only permissive, they also often use material rewards to try to keep their children in a constant state of happiness which, as we know, is rarely successful in the longer term.

And, finally, *uncaring* parents are low on both warmth and control. In this neglectful or chaotic style of parenting, it's easier to give in to the child's demands to keep them happy in the moment than to set healthy consistent limits which may take time to negotiate and understand. In this type of family the child is adrift without the support of secure attachments to their parents. The formation of their emerging personality can too easily become abnormal and their mental health is likely to suffer.

In summary the preferred style of *warm and respectful* parenting is:[4]

- **Nurturing:** Loving parental involvement makes a child more responsive to parental influence, creates a secure sense of self and a kind inner voice that enables them to socialise effectively and withstand the often harsh outside world.

4   Rowe, L., Bennett, D. and Tonge, B. (2009), *I Just Want You to be Happy: Preventing and Tackling Teenage Depression*, Sydney: Allen and Unwin.

- **Firm**: The combination of predictable support and clear limits helps with self-discipline. It allows the child to function as a responsible, competent individual, reduces exposure to risk and protects them from harmful, damaging experiences.
- **Autonomy granting**: The negotiation of rights and responsibilities at appropriate ages through the journey of adolescence allows for a healthy independence, at the same time fostering social cohesion and strong connections with peers and community.

DEALING WITH PARTNER SEPARATION

Every relationship has a beginning, a middle and an end.
A wise person celebrates where their relationship is.

Dr Ronald McCoy, contemporary doctor and philosopher

Separation and divorce are among some of the most difficult experiences anyone can have. Most people survive separation and go on to live happy and fulfilling lives. Unfortunately about half the people who remarry end up divorcing again. For this reason, it may be a good idea to consider seeking professional support and to attend partnering and parenting courses following separation.

Separation may not only mean loss of a partner, but loss of time with children and extended family, loss of the family home and neighbourhood, loss of friends and social life, and loss of meaning and hopes for the future. It is natural to grieve over these losses. It takes time to rebuild lives and social networks. For this reason it is common to experience depression and it is important to seek support, maintain a healthy lifestyle, avoid drugs and alcohol and try to continue normal routines and activities such as sport.

TIPS FOR DEALING WITH SEPARATION

- Don't hang onto the false hope that the original relationship will be restored but try to rebuild a different relationship with your ex-partner, especially if children are involved.
- Take responsibility for your own life and try not to blame others. Avoid self-pity and revenge.
- Seek counselling from a trusted professional as family and friends may find it difficult to discuss the details of your relationship breakdown.
- Try to work out residence and contact arrangements for your children amicably and consider grandparents and other extended family in these arrangements. Consider formal family mediation if you are having problems agreeing to these arrangements.
- Try to negotiate child support payments and property settlement.
- Consider undertaking a parenting course to deal with the special challenges of being a single or separated parent.

The support and nurture we derive from strong relationships with our partners, our family members and our friends can enable us to continue our roles as effective health care providers to our patients and our communities.

Just as we advise our patients about their relationships, so too we need to pay attention to our own relationships and seek support and guidance from friends and professional peers at times of need.

CHAPTER 7

OUR RELATIONSHIPS WITH OUR COLLEAGUES

Honour and shame from no condition rise.
Act well your part—there all the honour lies.

Alexander Pope (1688–1744), poet

Many doctors enjoy very close professional and personal relationships with peers. Strong bonds of friendship are often developed throughout medical school and specialist training programs with medical and other colleagues. We can provide each other with great mutual support and look out for each other.

On the negative side, the pressure to work excessive hours can create relationship difficulties with employers, supervisors, hospital administrators, practice partners and other colleagues.

It is worth noting the enormous variability in responses to strong personalities. One doctor may react negatively to a colleague's challenging behaviour and another may find it enriching to be challenged. For this reason, this chapter focuses on constructive ways of dealing with problem solving, conflict resolution and bullying.

TAKING CRITICISM PERSONALLY

Patient management is complex. It is often very easy to be critical of a colleague's management in a second opinion or in retrospect. For this reason, criticism by peers is very common in medical practice. Even well-meaning criticism can be difficult to listen to when we are already stressed.

Hopefully, all of us will have colleagues who are *critical* friends. Critical friends are those colleagues who give us constructive feedback within a trusting relationship. This is a part of continuous self-improvement.

In reality many of us do not react well to criticism. Sometimes we fear medico-legal implications and formal patient complaints. Sometimes it bruises our egos. But mainly we don't react well because we tend to work in isolation and have received very little training on how to deal with criticism.

TIPS FOR RESPONDING TO PERSONAL CRITICISM

- Remain gently assertive and calm. Try: 'Thank you for the feedback', 'I can see we both want what is best in this situation', 'I appreciate that you have high standards.'
- Acknowledge that people have the right to be critical but not to personalise the criticism. Try: 'When you are willing to treat me with respect, I will be open to listening to what you have to say.'
- If the criticism is vague, ask for specific examples so that you can understand the issue better. Try: 'Thanks for raising these issues so that we can talk about some solutions.'
- Show the person you understand the criticism by restating what the other person has said in their words. Try: 'I can see why you would be upset over this.', 'I understand and I'll bear that in mind in the future.'

- If you believe that the personal criticism is not justified, say so and explain why. Try 'I am not used to being personally attacked and I'll discuss this with you when you are ready to communicate calmly.'

TIPS FOR GIVING CRITICISM

- When you have the need to criticise the actions of others it may help to begin the conversation with non-threatening statements like: 'I hope that we can create a trusting relationship where we can give each other constructive feedback' or 'Could we talk about...'
- Then ask open questions to help identify the issue and work towards a solution.
- Focus on the behaviour not the person.
- Avoid personal attacks.
- Ask: 'Do you know why this happened? How can we work together to prevent this happening again?'

RECOGNISE CONFLICT AS AN OPPORTUNITY

Honest differences are often a healthy sign of progress.

Gandhi (1869–1948)

Conflict is an important part of interacting with other people. Conflict can be due to a communication failure or due to real personal differences. Mistaking one for the other can have serious consequences.

Dealing with conflict in an angry or emotional manner can be destructive. Avoiding conflict by non-assertiveness can be even more destructive as tensions fester. By failing to express our own opinions and needs, we can place ourselves in a situation where we may begin to perceive we are being treated unfairly or bullied.

There are many reasons why we avoid conflict. We may suffer from low self-esteem and doubt our own judgment. As children our parents may have squashed our confidence with negative messages when we disagreed with them. We may be too tired or too busy to take the time to address conflict. We learn to suppress our own feelings in interactions with patients and we may fall into this habit with our colleagues as well.

But conflict is a very common issue in our everyday lives. If we recognise conflict as an opportunity to build stronger relationships, we tend to deal with it more constructively.

TIPS FOR DEALING WITH CONFLICT MORE EFFECTIVELY

- Remain calm and appropriately assertive.
- Acknowledge any strong feelings on either side.
- Listen to understand, without interrupting. Understand the other person's intentions. What is really behind the conflict? What are their motivations?
- When you state your views, ask that the other person maintain a level of mutual respect by not interrupting you.
- Agree on trying to find an outcome that you can both support. This may require compromise by everybody.
- Be clear on the issues that you cannot compromise on.
- Establish the facts of the situation to ensure there is no misunderstanding.
- Be prepared to allow the other person to express frustration but be ready to terminate the meeting if discussions become irrationally angry.
- After an outcome has been agreed, contact the other person in a few days either with a written report of the meeting or a telephone call to thank them for the meeting and to ensure there is an agreed understanding of any outcomes.

TIPS FOR NEGOTIATING A CONFLICT

- Identify issues behind the conflict and why there is disagreement.
- List all the possible solutions to the conflict including the ones you can't agree on.
- Examine all the advantages and disadvantages of each solution.
- Together find a compromise to come up with the best solution.
- Implement the solution and review it later to determine if it is working for everyone.

DISCRIMINATION, HARASSMENT AND BULLYING[1]

To sin by silence when they should protest, makes cowards out of good men.

Abraham Lincoln (1809–1865)

Like any other members of the community we must uphold human rights and speak out against discrimination. We are advocates for our patients and we should be vigilant in our workplaces in ensuring discrimination does not occur.

In stressful work environments, many younger doctors report experiencing discrimination, harassment and bullying. As a professional group we must work to prevent these unacceptable practices.

1   The Discrimination, Harassment and Bullying Policy of The Royal Australian College of General Practitioners 2005.

WHAT IS DISCRIMINATION?

Discrimination includes direct discrimination and indirect discrimination. Direct discrimination occurs if another person is treated less favourably than others because of a personal characteristic such as gender, disability or sexuality.

Indirect discrimination occurs if a requirement, benefit, condition or practice is imposed that treats everyone in the same way and appears neutral, but which significantly reduces the ability of people with a particular personal characteristic to comply with or benefit from it.

WHAT IS HARASSMENT?

Harassment is any uninvited, unwelcome behaviour, which a reasonable person could anticipate would create intimidation, humiliation or offence for the other person in those particular circumstances.

Examples of harassment may include:

- Unwanted physical contact
- Offensive verbal comments
- Offensive jokes
- The display of offensive material
- Ostracism by an individual or group
- Mockery through ridicule, name calling or insulting or dismissive gestures
- Denigrating another person by means of rumour based on hearsay
- Any other behaviour that creates an unpleasant working environment

Sexual harassment is one form of harassment. Examples of sexual harassment include any act, behaviour or material of a sexual nature, including:

- Any act of unwanted physical closeness
- Jokes with sexual connotations
- Making promises or threats in return for sexual favours

- Displays of sexually graphic material including posters, cartoons or messages left on notice boards, desks, computer screens or common areas
- Propositions
- Lewd gestures
- Repeated invitations to go out after prior refusal
- Sex-based insults, taunts, the spreading of rumours, teasing or name calling
- Unwelcome physical contact such as massaging a person without invitation or deliberately brushing up against them
- Sexually explicit conversations
- Offensive phone calls, voicemails, letters, emails or text messages or computer screen savers

Behaviour that is based on mutual attraction, friendship and respect does not constitute sexual harassment. However, a previously consensual sexual relationship does not confer the right to sexual behaviour that is no longer welcome.

Stalking, sexual assault or rape are criminal activities and must be reported to the police.

WHAT IS BULLYING?

Workplace bullying is repeated, unreasonable behaviour directed towards an employee or volunteer that creates a risk to health and safety. The following types of behaviour, where repeated or occurring as part of a pattern of behaviour, could be considered bullying:

- Verbal abuse
- Excluding or isolating an individual
- Psychological harassment (e.g. isolating someone by preventing others from befriending them)
- Intimidation
- Derogatory comments
- Assigning meaningless tasks unrelated to the job
- Giving employees impossible assignments
- Deliberately changing work rosters to inconvenience particular individuals

- Constant criticism
- Suppression of ideas
- Deliberately withholding information that is vital for effective work performance
- Spreading rumours about an individual or group

Workplace bullying is about the bully's controlling needs and the focused and systematic selection of targets. Bullies are often oblivious to their actions and therefore a policy won't work in practice and the problem will not stop unless it is brought to their attention that they are behaving inappropriately.

In recent years, workplaces have become more aware of the need to be assertive in performance managing staff who repeatedly display bullying behaviours. This can particularly be the case where the perpetrator inflicts fear and feelings of extreme confusion and powerlessness in other people. On the surface the perpetrator may be charming and intelligent; however, they often lack insight into their bullying behaviour. The people who are being bullied are often not believed at first and may be labelled as weak or negative. Others often recognise the perpetrator's behaviour but prefer to stay neutral to avoid the risk of being targeted themselves. An organisation must not condone these behaviours whatever their motivation. Individual lives and organisations can be seriously damaged by inaction.

WHAT IS VICARIOUS LIABILITY?

Vicarious liability means that an employer may be found to be liable for the discrimination, harassment or bullying of others by its employees. It is the responsibility of employers to ensure a workplace free of discrimination, harassment and bullying.

If a complaint is made, the following principles apply:

- Offer support to anyone who is being discriminated against, harassed or bullied and advise them how to seek assistance.
- Deal promptly with any issue or complaint raised.
- As far as possible maintain the confidentiality of the people involved in a complaint of discrimination, harassment, bullying.

COMPLAINT RESOLUTION PROCEDURE

Organisations have a legal responsibility to ensure that their workplace is safe and free of discrimination, harassment and bullying. All doctors must be aware of basic safe work policies.

TIPS FOR DEALING WITH DISCRIMINATION, HARASSMENT OR BULLYING

Here are some steps to take if you have experienced discrimination, harassment or bullying:

- Document the evidence of the discrimination, harassment or bullying.
- Write a formal letter of complaint detailing the facts to the appropriate and most senior person in the workplace, which is usually the chief executive officer, human resources officer or the practice principal.
- The letter of complaint must be treated with the utmost confidentiality to protect the rights of the victim and the alleged perpetrator.
- It is the responsibility of the person who receives the formal complaint to meet separately with the person making the complaint and the alleged perpetrator to establish the facts.
- If the evidence is clear, an apology must be offered by the perpetrator, in a face-to-face meeting with the victim and the most senior officer of the organisation.
- The organisation or practice must ensure that the person who has made the complaint and other staff are not subjected to recurrences of discrimination, harassment or bullying. This can be done by revising policies and procedures and providing mandatory training to staff on bullying and harassment.

Our professional colleagues can provide us with great support in our role as doctors. Conflict is common in medical workplaces but it can be managed in a constructive way which benefits the care we provide to our patients. Bullying and discrimination are never acceptable behaviours.

CHAPTER 8

OUR RELATIONSHIP
WITH OUR PATIENTS

The essential unit of medical practice is the occasion when, in the intimacy of the consulting room, a person who is ill or believes himself to be ill seeks the advice of a doctor whom he trusts. This is a consultation and all else in the practice of medicine derives from it.

James Calvert Spence (1892–1954), paediatrician and researcher

Any doctor can become an excellent medical technician with the right training and experience. What sets a doctor apart in their patients' eyes is whether they are caring and kind as well as competent. For example, many patients would be critical if a surgeon bluntly delivers a poor prognosis related to a pathology result, even after performing a technically brilliant surgical operation. Our patients quite rightly expect more from us than medical interventions and technical expertise.

As doctors, we must also be mindful of the special needs of certain groups of patients who may be marginalised and discriminated against by their own communities. Often, their doctor may be the only person someone feels they can completely trust and confide in. For example, elderly people may require extra time to ensure they can make informed choices, people with a disability may require special attention to access and communication, and people from culturally and linguistically diverse backgrounds may require increased sensitivity to cultural beliefs about health and treatment. We need to be aware that we are a very important person in our patients' lives.

In theory, all doctors would agree with these principles. In reality, it is much harder to uphold a caring approach to all patients, particularly in a crowded public health care setting or towards patients we perceive to be challenging. It's easy to forget what it means to be kind in the process of juggling all the complex demands of patient care.

We also need to be mindful of the stresses faced by our staff which may result in negative interactions with our patients. This is a common cause of patient dissatisfaction and may be a source of complaints. It is worth taking time to observe what is really happening in our waiting rooms and on our front desk telephones. Staff training on basic customer service is especially important in a medical context where patients can be sensitive and fearful.

Sometimes it is important simply to remind ourselves and our staff to take time to enjoy our work.

DISCOVERING AND REDISCOVERING THE JOY OF BEING A DOCTOR

In an article entitled 'Being a doctor', US physician Dr Faith Fitzgerald[1] encouraged doctors to be caring and curious about their patients' stories in a therapeutic way and to ask patients to tell them more about themselves. She recounts the time she asked a junior doctor to choose a patient on the hospital ward he considered to be uninteresting. He chose an elderly woman out of compassion as she was in hospital because she had been evicted from her house and had nowhere else to go.

Dr Fitzgerald wrote, 'This woman had no real medical history but was simply suffering from the depredations of antiquity and abandonment and she was monosyllabic in her responses and gave a history of no substantive content. Nothing it seemed had ever

1   Fitzgerald, F. (1999), 'Being a doctor', *Annals of Internal Medicine*, 130: 70–72.

really happened to her. She had lived a singularly unexciting life as a hotel maid.'

Dr Fitzgerald then asked the woman how long she had lived in San Francisco and her answers went like this:[2]

Years and years.

Was she there for the earthquake?
No she came after.

Where did she come from?
Ireland.

When did she come?
1912

Had she ever been in hospital before?
Once

How did that happen?
Well she had broken her arm.

How had she broken her arm?
A trunk fell on it.

A trunk?
Yes.

What kind of trunk?
A steamer trunk.

How did that happen?
The boat lurched.

The boat?
The boat carrying her to America.

Why did the boat lurch?
It hit an iceberg.

Oh, what was the name of the boat?
The *Titanic*.

2   Fitzgerald, F. (1999), 'Being a doctor', *Annals of Internal Medicine*, 130: 70–72.

The elderly woman had been a passenger on the *Titanic* and was no longer uninteresting. Few of us have known patients who were passengers on the *Titanic*, but we can all recount these kinds of magic moments in medicine when the ordinary becomes the extraordinary and the story behind the history unfolds. In a time of increasing medical workforce shortage and time pressures, it can be difficult for doctors to remain curious about their patients' stories.

As Dr Faith Fitzgerald concluded:

> I believe it is our duty as those who teach young physicians to identify medical students with a gift for curiosity and take infinite pains to encourage that gift. Not only will patient care be enriched, but so will the lives of these physicians and the vigor of our art and science. Besides it will be much more interesting.[3]

DEALING WITH DIFFICULT CONSULTATIONS

In reality, there are many patients who challenge us in many different ways. It is difficult to be all things to all patients. However, there are ways of maintaining empathy for the patients we may find challenging while at the same time avoiding compassion fatigue.

THE PATIENT WITH A LIST

The person who presents with a long list of symptoms and high expectations is a common frustration for many doctors. We are all familiar with the person who comes in with a shopping list of complaints and who is unwilling to hand over the list but wishes to go through each point in detail one at a time. This may lead us to become frustrated because of limited time for the consultation or because we feel we are losing control of the consultation. However,

3 Fitzgerald, F. (1999), 'Being a doctor', *Annals of Internal Medicine*, 130: 70–72.

it is likely that this person has taken care to detail the health care concerns which are important to them. A patient with a list has often experienced past frustration with being rushed or feeling uncomfortable and out of control. The list may be a sign of excessive anxiety and fear. Alternatively the preparation of a list may signal a well-motivated person who is well prepared for the consultation and who wishes to participate in their own health care. This needs to be respected and the consultation managed in a way that does not leave the patient or the doctor frustrated.

If a patient presents with a long list of complaints or tasks, try to refrain from taking the list as this may be perceived by the patient as offensive. Ask them to read the full list up front to check if there are any urgent symptoms and work out with the patient the order of priority and whether there is any possible connection between symptoms. Then agree with the patient what can be done today and what needs to be deferred to a future appointment. A collaborative, respectful approach usually works best.

SOMATISATION

People who present repeatedly with unexplained physical symptoms such as chronic headaches, dizziness, palpitations or other aches and pains may have somatisation. This may be a sign of underlying depression and anxiety.

Ordering one more test or one more referral to satisfy the patient's conviction that there is something seriously wrong can be counterproductive. Implying that the symptoms are all in the mind can be just as ineffective.

In this situation it is important to take time to understand the person's concerns. It is usually helpful to make the connection between physical and mental disorders by using examples well known to patients, such as when a person develops nervous diarrhoea or palpitations or shortness of breath before a high school examination or an interview. We can reassure the patient that the symptoms are likely to resolve with treatment of underlying anxiety or depression and that they don't need to have physical symptoms in order to consult us.

ABNORMAL ILLNESS BEHAVIOUR

Abnormal illness behaviour is apparent when there are non-anatomical or behavioural descriptions of symptoms and unusual behavioural responses to physical examination. Beliefs, distress and illness behaviour can be powerful influences on pain. Illness behaviour can reflect a serious physical problem, but may be related more to psychological processes than to the underlying physical problem. For this reason, patients displaying illness behaviour often require specialist pain management and psychological interventions.

It is very difficult to manage patients with abnormal illness behaviour in isolation. A team approach is often essential for good patient care.

RESPONDING TO GRIEF AND LOSS

One of the most uplifting experiences in medicine is to witness patients and their families endure enormous suffering with courage and dignity. Stories of the way people respond to loss are sometimes inspirational.

Loss is not only felt with death, disability and loss of independence, but with other life changes such as relationship changes due to separation or divorce, job changes, particularly due to unemployment or retirement, change of role when children are born or leave home, or change of residence and moving away from family and friends. Grief and anger can be normal reactions in these circumstances, but when these feelings become entrenched or have a negative impact on wellbeing, they may lead to depression. As doctors, we can assist our patients manage grief and loss by encouraging them to deal with stress, maintain a healthy lifestyle and stay connected to family and friends.

We also help patients by empathising with their situation. Patients appreciate doctors who take time to listen and communicate concern. They also appreciate doctors who are comfortable with expressing their own emotions. It is natural and not uncommon for us to express emotion and to cry in response to the suffering of our patients.

DEALING EFFECTIVELY WITH PATIENT ANGER

Many patients become angry. This may be in response to a diagnosis, rudeness from members of staff, the length of waiting times, an adverse event, fear, grief or a perceived lack of support from family and friends. As doctors, we often bear the brunt of patient anger, and we need to learn how to react without taking this personally. When a patient is angry or a patient arouses anger in us, it is important to stand back from the situation, consider the underlying cause and remain calm.

Patient anger is often completely justifiable. It may relate to a past negative experience in another health service or in relation to another doctor. A calm question like: 'I sense you are angry. Can you tell me what is happening?' will often diffuse the situation and help our patients deal with very significant issues.

Active listening skills are important. Statements such as 'That must be very difficult for you', 'I am sorry you are feeling like this', 'What can I do to support you?' can often help to dissipate a patient's anger.

PEOPLE WITH PERSONALITIES WE FIND CHALLENGING

Sometimes patients with specific personality types are more likely to display anger and frustration because they feel misunderstood and they are unable to communicate their needs assertively. Here are a few examples of common personality types:

- A person who is preoccupied with details may have a tendency to be rigid and only undertake treatment with excessive cautiousness.
- A person who is hypersensitive to disapproval may have difficulty presenting for health care because of their fear of negative evaluation or rejection.
- A person who has a strong need for reassurance may have a tendency to seek frequent consultations.
- A person who displays a lack of emotional responsiveness may be reluctant to talk about their problems.

In all these cases it is likely that people will respond to active listening by us, and the provision of appropriate information and reassurance. Sometimes it is important to establish clear boundaries. Sometimes it may take longer to develop a trusting relationship. Nevertheless, taking time to understand the person as well as their illness is important in establishing a meaningful long-term therapeutic relationship. We are consistently surprised to discover that people who initially challenge us through their behaviour can teach us a great deal about what it means to be human and can become welcome visitors to our consulting rooms.

And never forget that people with challenging personalities can still experience real physical and mental illness. Someone with an obsessive personality can suffer real anxiety if their world doesn't match their world view and this can lead to depression. People with symptoms of hypochondria can still get sick and often experience higher rates of morbidity and mortality due to delays in diagnosis. We must never compromise the medical care of our patients who we may perceive to have challenging personalities or behaviours.

In the words of Sir William Osler, the best-known physician in the English-speaking world in the early 1900s, 'the consultation requires the art of equanimity which is a detachment of personal feelings and distractions; the virtue of using a systematic method for organised work; the quality of thoroughness in assessing symptoms, signs and opinions; the grace of humility; and a reverence for responsibility'.

RESPONDING TO A PATIENT COMPLAINT OR AN ADVERSE EVENT

One of the most stressful situations in medicine can be receiving a patient complaint or dealing with an adverse event. Those of us who have experienced medico-legal actions are more likely to practise more defensively after the experience and more likely to order investigations, refer to specialists, prescribe more medication and consider leaving clinical practice or retiring early. Those of us who have a current claim, complaint or critical incident are more likely to have a higher level of psychiatric illness and drink more alcohol.

A patient complaint or legal action is more likely if an adverse event has been handled insensitively, or there has been a delay in communication or poor communication after an incident. Open, honest, timely and caring communication is encouraged. Clearly, it is important to deal with complaints or adverse events effectively in order to restore trust in the doctor-patient relationship and prevent any risk of recurrence. People need to be reassured that their complaint is being taken seriously and responded to by the doctor concerned in a face to face meeting.

To mitigate against the risk of legal action, we are encouraged to contact our medical defence organisations immediately after a patient has made a complaint and before an apology is offered. Open disclosure is to be encouraged but must be undertaken in consultation with our medical defence organisation. If unintended clinical harm has occurred, it is appropriate for the treating doctor to:

- Establish the facts behind the complaint and the factors that led to the complaint, to deal with the patient's concerns and identify any changes that can be implemented to prevent this happening to another person. It may be helpful to provide this information to the patient.

- Communicate that an adverse event has occurred to the patient.

- Try to re-establish patient trust by having a face to face meeting. Use a concerned, sincere tone, take your time during the meeting and offer to work with the patient to address the situation together.

- Listen to the patient carefully and establish what the patient expects to happen after the complaint. Many people want to be reassured that this will not happen to another person and may seek compensation if this is the only way to raise awareness about the medical mishap. Others will take legal action to punish the doctor or to raise money.

- Validate the patient's anger by saying 'It must be very frustrating for you'.
- Express regret for what has happened by saying 'I am very sorry this has happened', 'I am upset about this outcome' without admitting negligence or error of judgment.
- Provide relevant clinical information and document the process of dealing with the complaint. Ask if there is anything else the patient needs to know about or if the patient requires any other support.
- Discuss appropriate ways of dealing with the payment of accounts. For example, it may be appropriate to waive payment. Do not send accounts for incorrect treatment.
- Provide options for ongoing medical care or referral.

Medical defence organisations will advise against making any admission of liability that proves negligence. For example, it is inadvisable to admit an incident was an error or an error of judgment. Expressions of sympathy do not constitute an admission of fault.

After any adverse event, it is important for a hospital or practice team to undertake root cause analysis to determine the cause and contributing factors, in order to prevent a similar incident affecting another patient. Sometimes this involves identifying clinical training needs and clinical guidelines, reviewing processes for obtaining consent and examining the systems that have contributed to failure such as complaints-handling processes, processes for reviewing results, infection control procedures, recruitment and training of staff and the management of confidentiality and privacy.

Doctors have become more aware of the importance of risk identification and management in everyday practice. While this can be a time-consuming process, most doctors understand the importance of doing this to prevent medical errors and improve the quality of clinical care.

PREVENTION AND MANAGEMENT OF PATIENT-INITIATED VIOLENCE[4]

Safety and security don't just happen: they are the result of collective consensus and public investment. We owe our children—the most vulnerable citizens in any society—a life free from violence and fear. In order to ensure this, we must become tireless in our efforts not only to attain peace, justice and prosperity for countries but also for the communities and members of the same family. We must address the roots of violence. Only then will we transform the past century's legacy from a crushing burden into a cautionary lesson.

Nelson Mandela (1918–)

As doctors, we are quick to recognise that patient anger is often justified and not directed at us personally. It is our role to mediate anger and to understand its underlying cause. Anger usually quickly dissipates when it is managed calmly. Occasionally patient anger escalates to become a personal threat against a doctor and we must recognise the point at which strong emotion tips into threatening behaviour. A threat of violence is never acceptable behaviour.

Patient-initiated violence is increasingly common in medical practice and is a reflection of increasing community violence. While zero tolerance is a superficially attractive proposition, most doctors find it ineffective in practice as it usually only deflects violent behaviour onto other colleagues or to the wider community. In medical practice, patients who display violent behaviours usually have an underlying disorder which requires assertive clinical management. For this reason medical workplace violence is underreported to police.

---

4   This section is adapted from Rowe, L., Morris-Donovan, B and Watts, I (2009), *General Practice: A Safe Place*, Melbourne: The Royal Australian College of General Practioners.

In assessing the severity of violence, we must examine the intention behind the threat. The definition of assault is any act which intentionally or recklessly causes another person to fear immediate and unlawful violence. Verbal threats of violence can be more damaging than unintended physical assault. For example, a threat by a patient to abduct our children from school is likely to be more harmful than an accidental punch in the face from a patient in extreme pain.

The effects of patient-initiated violence are serious for doctors and other staff and include anxiety, depression, stress-related illness, diminished productivity due to poor concentration, social withdrawal and reduced participation in the medical workforce.

Patient-initiated violence is an occupational health and safety issue. It is an issue that needs to be managed by identifying:

- the extent and nature of the risk
- the factors that contribute to the risk
- the changes necessary to eliminate or control the risk and
- monitoring and evaluation of the risk-control process.

Doctors and other medical staff must feel confident expressing anxieties regarding patient behaviour. The hospital or medical practice must not accept threatening behaviour as a 'normal' way of working or as 'just part of the job'. Staff must be reassured that their concerns will be acted on.

When confronting an angry person who is threatening violence, and especially when we are about to ask someone to leave, it can be

SOME BASIC TIPS FOR DE-ESCALATING AGGRESSIVE BEHAVIOUR

- Appear calm, respectful, self-controlled and confident.
- Use reflective questioning where you can. For example: 'You need to see a doctor as soon as possible, is that correct?'
- Use a neutral tone and offer to help: 'I'd like to help you.'
- Use neutral body language.
- Embrace silence.

useful to invite an observer into the room. They don't say anything but their presence will often defuse a potentially violent situation.

In medical practice the prevention of patient-initiated violence is dependent on the identification and assertive clinical management of patients at risk. This may include people with:

- Borderline Personality Disorder
- Alcohol and drug problems
- Untreated psychosis.

It must be emphasised that many people with these problems are more likely to be the victims rather than the perpetrators of violence. People with mental illness often experience very damaging stigma and discrimination in the community and no one wants to add to this situation. Nevertheless, there are times when people with untreated disorders lose control of their ability to regulate their emotions and doctors have a responsibility to manage threatening behaviours assertively and to ensure that their patients are not at risk of harm to themselves or to others.

Unfortunately people with mental illness and drug and alcohol problems are over-represented in the criminal justice system. This is a human rights issue directly related to poor access to comprehensive mental health care in the community.

BORDERLINE PERSONALITY DISORDER

Borderline Personality Disorder is a psychiatric illness defined by DSM IV criteria as including five or more of the following symptoms that are pervasive over a range of social and personal situations:

- Frantic efforts to avoid real or imagined abandonment
- Unstable and intense personal relationships
- Impulsivity in at least two self-destructive ways including excessive spending, gambling, sex, abuse of alcohol, use of other drugs, dangerous driving and road rage or binge eating
- Recurrent threats of self-harm, self-mutilation or suicidal behaviour
- Mood changes
- Chronic feelings of emptiness

- Difficulty controlling anger, temper and violent behaviour
- Transient stress-related paranoia or dissociative symptoms.

This disorder is a disorder of regulation of emotions and affects about 2% of people, especially young women. The disorder is thought often to be related to neglect and physical and emotional abuse as children or negative stressful events in adolescence.

People with Borderline Personality Disorder are sensitive to rejection and usually react with anger to mild disturbances. They are often seen by doctors as a result of being harmed through their destructive behaviours.

Group and individual psychotherapy and pharmacological treatments can be effective. Doctors can help a patient with Borderline Personality Disorder by scheduling regular appointment times with the same health care professional, and encouraging the patient to follow a daily routine. Setting limits on destructive behaviours can be helpful.

People with Borderline Personality Disorder are more likely to be the victims rather than the perpetrators of violence, often at their own hand. Their impulsive behaviours can bring them into dangerous situations or relationships. People with Borderline Personality Disorder sometimes target their doctor with destructive and violent behaviours and require assertive clinical management, which may require the involvement of the police.

PEOPLE WITH ALCOHOL AND DRUG PROBLEMS

Those of us who have been in practice for a number of years will have seen many people who have come through drug or alcohol addiction and go on to lead happy and productive lives. It is important to remain open to assisting people who are pre-contemplative or contemplative about reducing alcohol or drug use.

It can be difficult to determine the difference between someone who is genuinely seeking help and someone who may be misrepresenting the truth to obtain drugs of addiction. A comprehensive history and examination can help shed more light on the person's

BEHAVIOUR CONTRACT

It may be useful to have a behaviour contract for patients who have exhibited unacceptable behaviour in our practices or hospitals. This example of a behaviour contract should be tailored to the particular situation.[5]

Acceptable behaviour contract

I,_____(patient) agree to a contract with
_____(hospital/practice)

As part of this contract I will not

- Shout, yell or make a loud noise which disturbs others.
- Make verbal or physical threats.
- Attend intoxicated.
- Damage or steal property.
- Follow staff or doctors.

Should I breach this contract I understand that:

I may be asked to leave this hospital/practice,

Police attendance may be requested, and

My future attendance at this hospital/practice may be prohibited and I may have to seek health care elsewhere.

Declaration: I confirm that I understand the meaning of this contract and the consequences of breach of the contract have been explained to me.

Signed: Date:
Witness: Date:

---

5   Associate Professor Moira Sim (2008), The Obsorne GP Network website on medical
    workplace violence, <www.snmpm.ecu.edu.au/research/aggression>, viewed 8 May
    2009.

motivation. Patients who are genuinely seeking assistance will usually cooperate fully with this approach. Patients who are only seeking a prescription will often leave after the first few questions although some can be very persistent.

If we ever feel threatened by a patient, especially someone who appears to be affected by alcohol or drugs and is seeking a prescription or needles, we should consider giving the patient what they want and asking them to leave immediately. If we do this, we must then report our actions to the police.

PATIENTS WITH UNTREATED PSYCHOSIS

Unfortunately people with psychosis are overrepresented in the criminal justice system. About 10% of people who commit murder or major crime are acutely psychotic at the time of the incident. Tragically, many of these people have fallen through the gaps in our mental health systems and end up receiving mandatory treatment in the criminal justice system.

For this reason, acute psychosis, especially first-onset schizophrenia, should be treated as a medical emergency. Schizophrenia has a better lifetime prognosis if treated with antipsychotic medication early, usually within one week of the development of acute symptoms. Delays in treatment may result in lifelong disability or death by suicide or occasionally by police.

It is important for people with treated psychosis to establish a strong relationship with their treating doctor and other supporting health care providers. Education and support of the patient and their family and friends are essential for a good outcome.

Patients who are a risk to themselves and/or others may require supported, emergency involuntary admission to hospital.

REVIEWING AN INCIDENT OF MEDICAL WORKPLACE VIOLENCE

Any incident of patient-initiated violence should be reviewed. Whether it occurred in a hospital, in a private medical practice or on a home visit, doctors must meet with members of their team to discuss the following questions:

- What happened?
- What factors may have triggered the violence?
- Could the incident have been prevented?
- How should we manage this patient now?
- What safeguards or barriers can be put in place to minimise the risk of recurrence?
- Have the police been informed and what advice was received?

These questions not only assist medical staff members to manage the current situation but help prevent future episodes. Often staff members can identify ways to create a safer physical environment. In the case of major violence, it may be necessary to terminate the doctor–patient relationship.

SAFE PHYSICAL ENVIRONMENTS

We all have a responsibility to both our patients and the members of our staff to ensure that the physical environments of our hospitals and clinics are safe for everybody. However, changes to our physical environments must be considered in the context of patient access. For example, wider and higher counters at reception minimise the ability of patients to lean over the counter and physically harm a receptionist, but may limit communication with reception staff for a patient with disability.

Here are some practical tips for creating safer physical environments:

- Create physical barriers between the waiting area and the consulting rooms to prevent unauthorised access by patients to working areas. Most modern businesses have a barrier to prevent clients entering consulting rooms without a staff member to protect the security of staff, cash, personal and practice property and confidential documents.
- Install security locks on all windows and access doorways.
- Lock the back doors and lock all consulting rooms whenever they are empty.
- Glass in all windows and doors should be shatter-proof.

- Consider removing any pictures in the public areas with non-shatter-proof glass as the glass can be broken and used as a weapon.
- Waiting room and consulting room signs should be prominently displayed notifying that cash is not kept on site and drugs of addiction are not prescribed by the practice.
- The chairs in consulting rooms can be arranged so that the doctor or other treating health professional is always sitting closest to the door. However, many professionals recognise that it may be better to give their patients easy access to the door to allow the patient to leave if they become agitated.
- Install effective lighting in corridors, car parks, walkways and the external surrounds of buildings.
- Erect fencing to prevent the practice grounds and car park being used as a public thoroughfare.
- Install duress alarms and ensure there is an agreed staff policy in place to respond when an alarm is activated and ensure that drills are held on a regular basis to test the adequacy of the response.
- Maintain a practice policy of never allowing a staff member to be alone on the premises at times when the practice is open to patients.
- Hospital and medical practice staff may also find it helpful to have a code of conduct that can be handed to patients who display unreasonable anger to make them aware of their responsibilities.

HOME VISIT POLICY

Home visits can be an integral part of the care of some patients, particularly the terminally ill or the frail and elderly. However, the safety of the attending doctor must always be considered. Home visits should not be provided without triaging the patient to assess their need for a home visit. Where possible, patient files should be flagged to ensure staff are warned if they are likely to be unwelcome at the home, or if the patient or other residents at the address have a known history of violence. Consider whether home visits without the use of an accompanying person for appropriate security are appropriate.

CODE OF CONDUCT[6]

This practice/hospital aims to provide a safe and pleasant environment for all patients and staff. We ask everyone who attends this practice/hospital to follow this Code of Conduct.

This Code of Conduct states that everyone should behave in a way that respects the dignity and rights of others.

The following behaviour falls outside the Code of Conduct and is therefore unacceptable.

- Shouting or loud noise which disturbs others
- Offensive remarks
- Threatening or aggressive remarks, gestures or actions
- Intoxication
- Damage to property
- Theft
- Physical assault

Unacceptable behaviour will have consequences. You may have services limited and you may not be allowed to return to the practice/hospital.

Violent behaviour is never tolerated and the police will be called.

- Do not agree to home visits to patients threatening suicide or domestic violence or who are aggressive in their language without involving the police.
- Advise unfamiliar patients to come to the practice or attend an emergency department for specific pain relief medication or repeat prescriptions.
- Keep a record at the practice of the registration, make, model and colour of all doctors' cars.

6   Associate Professor Moira Sim (2008), The Osborne GP Network website on medical workplace violence, <www.snmpm.ecu.edu.au/research/aggression>, viewed 8 May 2009

- Always walk on the best lit side of the street, stay away from bushes and parks.
- If driving, check the back seat before unlocking the vehicle and park pointing the exit to allow an easy escape.
- If there is a lift stand by the control panel to control the lift and have quick access to the alarm.
- Ensure procedures are in place and followed if staff cannot be contacted or do not return or check back in as expected.
- If using a deputising service, it must be alerted regarding any patients who may be at high risk of being violent.

STALKING

Stalking is more common than we think. Stalking is a pattern of repeated, unwanted attention, harassment and contact that causes the victim to believe that the offender (stalker) will cause them physical harm or that the offender wants to cause them mental distress. Stalking should be recognised early so that it may be dealt with promptly and effectively. Every medical workplace should have in place a policy which informs staff how to protect themselves.

TIPS FOR DEALING WITH STALKING

- Document every contact with the stalker, including telephone calls, emails, letters and deliverables.
- Record all cases of being followed by car or on foot, or being watched. The documentation provides evidence that you have been stalked.
- Contact the police every time the stalker makes contact. The police should also maintain documentation. Ask for a copy of the police log.
- Request that the police assess the security of your practice.
- Have a phone with a caller-identification screen. Log all calls from the stalker, recording time, date and nature of the call, for example 'heavy breathing'.

- Advise the practice team, friends, family and neighbours of the situation. Ask people to watch for any unusual activity near your home, workplace or car.
- Keep the outside of your practice and home well lit and free of places where a stalker may hide.
- Install appropriate locks, deadlocks, window security, flood lights, security screens and door alarms in your practice and home.
- Considering filing a restraining order against the stalker through your solicitor.
- Never enter into a conversation with a stalker.
- Consider enrolling in a self-defence course.
- Vary your routines. For example, go home by different routes at different times and arrive at work at different times.
- Keep your car locked when you are driving.
- If you travel by public transport plan your trip to avoid excessive waiting times at bus or train stops. When stepping off a bus or train ensure you are not being followed.

At the same time a complaint about criminal conduct is made to the police, their assistance should be sought about taking out an intervention order and, if necessary, further legal advice should be sought.

TERMINATING PATIENT–DOCTOR RELATIONSHIPS

There are going to be times when it is necessary or wise to terminate the care of an individual patient. This may be related to violent or inappropriate behaviour by the patient or other occasions when the doctor is unable to continue to provide best possible care.

As with all aspects of clinical care, a thoughtful and considered approach, including clear communication, will help minimise any potential harm to the patient.

It is often wise to seek medico-legal advice when terminating a doctor—patient relationship.

In communicating the decision to terminate a therapeutic relationship, make every effort to ensure that the patient understands what is being said. It is usually better if the decision is communicated face to face, even if this is difficult.

If the reasons for terminating the relationship are sensitive, it might be appropriate to have another person present at the meeting. In some cases it might be best for another doctor in the practice to talk the patient through our decision. If telling the patient face to face is not possible, we should at least inform the patient of our decision in a sensitively written letter that explains that it is no longer possible for us to treat the patient. Patients should not be informed of our decision at the reception desk next to a crowded waiting room.

If the patient requires ongoing medical care, we should offer them a referral to another treating doctor. The patient's new doctor should be provided with enough information from the patient's medical file to enable ongoing care and to prevent the patient needing to submit to further tests and investigations unnecessarily. This might require photocopying the entire file or, if confidentiality is an issue, providing a summary of the file.

> *Medical practice is a great privilege and provides many examples of joy and inspiration throughout our career.*
>
> *At the same time medical practice is not without its challenges. Being prepared, cautious and aware can reduce the risk of harm to us in any challenging encounter.*

CHAPTER 9

OUR RELATIONSHIP WITH OUR PHYSICAL ENVIRONMENT

Climate change is one of the greatest challenges of our time. Climate change will affect, in profoundly adverse ways, some of the most fundamental determinants of health: food, air, water. In the face of this challenge, we need champions throughout the world who will work to put protecting human health at the centre of the climate change agenda.

Dr Margaret Chan, Director General of the World Health Organization

Our health and the health of our patients can be compromised by our physical environment. Medical workplaces have the well-deserved reputation for being physically unfriendly. Daily exposure to cramped cubicles, under-functioning or over-functioning air conditioning, fluorescent lights, grey walls and floors and a mix of unpleasant smells and excessive noise can be dehumanising. And unless we manage our own architect-designed private medical practice, it can be difficult to do anything about this.

Whether we work in a hospital or a medical clinic, each of us can bring to work reminders of what it is to be human. It is possible to personalise our space and reclaim offices and staff rooms with simple things like photos of family, artwork from our paediatric patients, plants, aromatherapy oils, music and bowls of fresh fruit.

YOUR POSTURE

At a personal level, one of the most basic of all physical needs is to have a comfortable chair and to be aware of your posture while working in your consulting room or at your computer.

- Ensure that you are comfortable when you are sitting.
- Your computer must be straight ahead with no neck bending.
- Your chair should support your lower back.
- Keep your wrists straight without resting them on the desk.
- The height of your chair should be such that you have relaxed shoulders with your elbows hanging by your sides.
- Clean your computer monitor regularly.
- Ensure you have optimal lighting.
- Take regular breaks.
- Regularly stretch your arms and fingers, rotate your shoulders, shrug your shoulders, shake your arms, stand up and stretch your arms and legs.
- Take a brisk walk when possible.
- Take meal breaks away from your work area.

At the same time it is important to consider making our hospitals and medical practices more environmentally friendly. There is growing awareness of the need for hospitals and other medical workplaces to reduce the use of non-renewable energy and non-recycled water, to recycle materials when possible and to ensure waste disposal is environmentally sound. The use of fresh air, natural lighting and solar panels are being considered in new medical buildings. Medical workplaces are recycling plastics, cardboard and other recyclable materials. There are also examples where hospitals are working with local councils to supply bicycle paths, storage racks for bikes and access to showers for staff and incentives for staff to use car pooling or take a bus to work.

a green practice

Here are some ideas to make your medical workplace more environmentally friendly.

Ten tips for a green medical clinic (developed by the Australian Conservation Foundation and Doctors for the Environment Australia)[1]

1. **Install low-energy lighting.**
   - Replace old-style incandescent globes with compact fluoro globes or use fluorescent tubes. Avoid halogen downlights.
   - Replacing one incandescent globe with a compact fluoro can save 0.5 tonne of greenhouse gas and save money in energy costs in its lifetime (about 8 years).

2. **Turn off computers and appliances to save energy.**
   - Turn off computers and screens when not in use.
   - Turn off standby power at the end of each day, that is, switch off all appliances at the wall or power board (e.g. photocopiers, printers, chargers).

3. **Buy 'green power' for your clinic.**
   - Ask your energy supplier to switch you to accredited green power, or change to another energy supplier with accredited green power.
   - Buying 100% green power means that all your electricity will come from wind, solar or other renewable sources.

4. **Use energy-efficient refrigerators.**
   - Aim to have the most energy efficient and smallest refrigerator(s) you can. When buying a refrigerator choose the one that uses the least energy per year.
   - Maintain your existing refrigerator(s) to be as efficient as possible:
     —ensure the seals are completely intact and gripping—replace any damaged ones;
     —position your refrigerator so that it has air space around it to expel the heat it generates (especially behind and above) and keep it away from the sun.

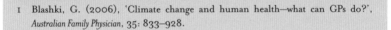

1   Blashki, G. (2006), 'Climate change and human health—what can GPs do?', *Australian Family Physician*, 35: 833–928.

5. Reduce car journeys.
   - Arrange pick-up with pathology companies in advance to avoid them making unnecessary trips—try to restrict pick-ups and deliveries to the minimum number per day.
   - Encourage staff to take public transport or ride to work—provide bicycle storage and changing facilities.
   - Reducing petrol usage from car trips saves greenhouse gases—with every litre of petrol saved 2.5 kg of greenhouse pollution is saved.

6. Aim for a paper-free office.
   - Communicate with doctors and patients by email where possible.
   - Request that test results and other information be sent to you by email.
   - Manage files and patient records on computer to avoid the need for printed documents.
   - When using paper for printing, try to reduce paper usage by printing on both sides of the page and only print the pages you need.

7. Recycle paper and plastics.
   - Arrange for a regular paper and plastic container recycling collection.
   - Have a paper shredder to shred patient documents before recycling.
   - Make the recycling bins available to both patients and staff and clearly label the recycling and landfill bins.

8. Buy recycled paper, stationery and toilet tissue.
   - Try to buy 50–100% recycled office paper.
   - Look for other stationery made from recycled materials (e.g. toners, pens, pencils).
   - Buy recycled toilet paper, kitchen towel and tissues.
   - Arrange for your toner cartridges to be collected for refill or recycling.

9. Save water in the bathroom and kitchen.
   - Fit aerators to all taps to reduce tap water usage by up to 50%.
   - Fix all dripping taps or leaking toilets immediately.
   - Convert an old single-flush toilet to a dual-flush toilet or install a cistern regulator which allows the user to determine the flush length.

10. Reduce junk mail.
    • Put a 'No junk mail' sticker on your letterbox.
    • Ask to be taken off the direct mail lists of pharmaceutical companies and other businesses who regularly post you materials you do not want.

The International Society of Doctors for the Environment (ISDE) aims to defend our environment both locally and globally to prevent numerous illnesses, ensure the necessary conditions for health and improve the quality of life. ISDE reinforces the need to care for the environment in order to safeguard the health of our own generation and of future generations. ISDE represents national organisations of medical practitioners in many countries.

> *A healthy physical environment is fundamental to good health.*
> *While we may have direct control over our immediate physical environment,*
> *we can also have a global impact through working with our colleagues*
> *and national and international organisations.*

CHAPTER 10

OUR RELATIONSHIP WITH OUR MEDICAL ORGANISATIONS

The art of medicine consists in amusing the patient while nature effects the cure.

Voltaire (1694–1778)

A natural death is where you die without the aid of a doctor.

Mark Twain (1835–1910)

I'm not feeling too well. I need a doctor immediately.
Quick, call the nearest golf course.

Groucho Marx (1890–1977)

My doctor gave me six months to live, but when I couldn't pay
the bill he gave me six months more.

Walter Matthau (1920–2000)

Not all of us find such jokes about doctors funny. But what we cannot ignore is that they reflect some long-entrenched community attitudes about doctors being poor communicators who may also be arrogant and appear uncaring. While these perceptions do not apply to us all, it often seems that we do very little to correct them.

In any business, falling customer satisfaction is a cause for concern. Many companies spend enormous amounts of time and money monitoring customer feedback and on branding and marketing to address consumer criticism and to change consumer attitudes. As doctors, our businesses are protected by medical workforce shortages, and we often do not appear to take customer criticism seriously. While there is an understandable reluctance on the part of doctors to advertise, it could be argued that our medical organisations have an important role in promoting the achievements of our profession on our behalf and in the interests of improving patient access to health care.

Many of us become concerned when we see public disunity between some of our medical organisations. The tendency for the media to focus on issues related to doctor remuneration and lack of accountability only strengthens the attitude that many doctors are working in their own interests, rather than for the public good. We know that this is not true.

There are many different organisations that represent the interests of medical practitioners and our patients. Membership of some organisations may be compulsory, for example the local medical practitioner board and medical indemnity or insurance provider. Membership of other medical organisations is voluntary and we need to consider which organisations we wish to support through our subscriptions.

While our diversity is one of our strengths as a profession, there are weaknesses associated with being represented by a complex and often fragmented system of medical organisations. Multiple newsletters and websites add to our information overload. We often feel we carry the burden related to patient care and professional standards alone. Yet our professional organisations exist to provide us with advocacy and support while ensuring that our patients have access to the highest quality health care.

There are many important professional issues that affect the day to day work of all doctors, and require strong advocacy by our medical organisations.

ACCESS TO CARE

Inequity in access to health services is a concern for many people. Chronic underfunding of primary care services, mental health services, drug and alcohol services, dental services and accident and emergency departments is a continuing source of frustration for many doctors and their patients.

Doctors who work in disadvantaged communities or with groups of vulnerable people face a daily struggle to deliver basic health services to their patients.

As an Australian example, child and adolescent psychiatrist, Professor Helen Milroy says this about the wider advocacy role of doctors and medical organisations in relation to Aboriginal disadvantage:

Doctors play a vital role in Aboriginal health as both practitioners and influential citizens. Unfortunately many doctors who work in Aboriginal communities find the challenge overwhelming and feel marginalised by other medical colleagues. Some of our Indigenous doctors find it hard to fight the inequity and discrimination still occurring with regard to Indigenous patients. This increases the complexity of roles doctors play. All doctors must understand the impact of historical legacy on disadvantage. Medical organisations must support doctors to meet these challenges.

QUALITY OF CARE

All doctors are concerned about ensuring that their patients have access to the highest possible level of quality medical care. Adverse events are often the result of failures in health care systems. Many of the most common and costly adverse events in hospitals and medical practices, including medication errors and hospital-acquired infections, can be prevented given appropriate resources and well-trained and supported staff.

CLINICAL INDEPENDENCE

The World Medical Association (www.wma.net) has affirmed 'the importance of professional autonomy and clinical independence, not only as an essential component of high quality medical care and therefore a benefit to the patient that must be preserved, but also as an essential principle of medical professionalism'.

Every day, doctors face considerable pressure from governments, health departments and health administrators seeking to influence clinical decision making, in ways which may not be in the best interests of our individual patients. Our medical organisations have a role in developing and disseminating evidence-based clinical guidelines which are based on research, rather than on restrictions enforced by inadequate funding.

ACCOUNTABILITY

As doctors, we of course need to be accountable for our clinical decisions and actions. Medical organisations must assist us to be aware of our obligations in relation to new government regulations and accreditation requirements. Keeping up to date with changes can be time consuming and complex and can add to our daily stress. Medical organisations can also assist governments and other non-government organisations seeking to improve ways to interact effectively with medical practitioners and so work together to improve the safety and quality of health care.

ADVOCACY

Our medical organisations should undertake root-cause analysis every time a catastrophic event occurs affecting a medical practitioner, such as a doctor dying by suicide or a doctor being seriously assaulted or killed in the course of their work. We cannot accept a continuation of doctors having a higher suicide rate than the general population or doctors and other health care providers being the victims of serious medical workplace violence. Our medical organisations should be involved in working together to monitor trends and implement systems which promote safe working environments.

There are many other issues that medical organisations are working on with governments, private health insurers, hospitals and organisations, including ethical dilemmas related to new technologies, e-health, health issues in the media and the threat of new and re-emerging diseases. The areas of concern appear endless and it is difficult for many medical organisations to communicate effectively the extent of their work to their members.

Few of us understand how to access support from our membership organisations about the issues that affect us. Few of us provide feedback to our medical organisations in response to surveys seeking member opinion. Although many medical organisations provide excellent support for their members, many of us do not utilise available services or have the time to visit our professional organisations' websites or read our organisations' publications to update ourselves on new initiatives and activities.

Medical organisations are only as strong as the support of their members. We recommend that all doctors consider making a contribution to a group or committee of at least one medical organisation. By being involved even in a limited way we gain peer support, have the opportunity to explore an area of special interest, diversify our professional activity and learn how our organisations work and how we can access future support. For example, by offering to join a clinical committee on an area of special interest, not only will we make a contribution to an issue we feel passionately about, but we may also meet senior doctors who could provide a mentoring role for us.

We believe that one of the most important roles of our medical organisations is to foster and train the next generation of medical leaders. Young doctors are the future of our profession and need to feel well engaged with our member organisations. There are times in each of our lives when we will be asked or feel the necessity to take on a leadership role. Leadership training and opportunities should be available to all doctors.

It is common for health issues to dominate elections of governments. As a united profession, doctors have considerable power and influence, especially when working with consumer advocacy organisations and bodies representing other health care professionals, in determining the priorities of key health issues affecting the people of the nation and in recommending workable solutions to address issues which affect the ability of patients to access high-quality medical and other health care services.

If we can't find the support we require for an issue of concern, we can write directly to the president or chair of our member organisation. The leaders of our medical organisations are accountable to the members of the organisations and we should expect a timely response to our letter and advice pointing us in the right direction. For many serious issues, often the leaders of an organisation will be hearing concerns expressed by a number of members. It is through members being vocal about their concerns that the leaders of medical organisations become aware of the urgency of key issues and the necessity for prompt advocacy and action.

If we don't engage with our member organisations we can't expect them to work effectively for us.

CHAPTER 11

DEALING WITH A MAJOR PERSONAL CRISIS

If you can meet with Triumph and Disaster
And treat those two imposters just the same...

Rudyard Kipling (1865–1936), from 'If'

As doctors, we are not immune from experiencing personal crisis. This is yet another reason why it is important to have our own trusted medical practitioner and to maintain strong relationships with our families and friends throughout our lives. While dealing with a major personal crisis can be devastating, many doctors have utilised the lessons learned through such an event to become even more effective clinicians and healers. However, some of us react by throwing ourselves into our work as a way of coping, which can be destructive in the long term.

In this chapter we outline four serious personal crises which we as doctors may face and reflect on what supports are available to assist us in a time of greatest need.

POST-TRAUMATIC STRESS DISORDER

I feel I should have sought crisis debriefing after my first patient death on the operating table. I spent months feeling that it was my fault (which it wasn't) and being terrified that every patient was going to lose blood and die. Compounding the problem was my junior status, my rural location and lack of consultant support. When the death occurred the consultant left the hospital immediately after telling me to close the abdomen and 'sort it out' with the family. I suspect mentoring, a supportive network and appropriate crisis debriefing would all have been helpful to me.

A general surgical registrar

It is common for members of the public to develop an acute stress reaction or a post-traumatic stress disorder in response to witnessing death or suicide or being involved in motor car accidents, medical emergencies, natural disasters, homicide, family violence, physical or sexual assault, stalking, threats, home invasion or property damage. Doctors can also experience stressful reactions to such events in the course of our work or personal lives. We may also be at risk of vicarious traumatisation after providing counselling and support to our patients who have experienced catastrophic events.

It can be difficult for us to take time away from our own practices to attend to our own distress. In our experience doctors working in rural and remote areas may experience even greater stress when responding to significant incidents as a result of often working in isolation, having to rely more on clinical skills rather than on investigations, and sometimes having inadequate or poorly maintained equipment and facilities. We often have prior knowledge of victims of traumatic events and may suffer self-recrimination and a burden of responsibility and also be exposed to possible sanctions from other community members, for example when resuscitation attempts have not been successful.

Acute stress disorder is defined as a short-term reaction to trauma which impairs a person's ability to function. It usually lasts between two days and four weeks. After experiencing an episode of trauma, it is a normal reaction to have cycling of strong emotion usually for about 10 days. The cycling often involves intrusive memories of the event and avoidance behaviour with associated numbness and denial.

To work through a traumatic experience, we encourage our patients to confront the memories of trauma, allow themselves to re-experience the thoughts, talk about the event and cry. It is also important to seek support from family and friends as this can help patients find meaning in the trauma and facilitate recovery. This is followed by a period of adjustment and time out when a sense of equilibrium and resilience is restored.

As doctors, however, we often do not have the ability to confide in family and friends about our personal reactions to a traumatic event especially if patient confidentiality is involved. We often don't take the time to attend debriefing or counselling. Instead of resting and taking time out after a highly stressful situation, we often have to cope with the community fallout following an incident.

In order to deal with the emergency at hand, we can risk delaying our own reaction to a traumatic event. However, ongoing depression, intense fear, nightmares and feelings of helplessness and horror cannot always be suppressed and may emerge as post-traumatic stress disorder. As doctors, we often underestimate the seriousness of this treatable condition. It is essential to seek professional help and incident debriefing.

THOUGHTS ABOUT SUICIDE

Depression has a major association with suicide because of the feelings of hopelessness, frustration and hostility. The explanation for the increased prevalence of suicide rates in doctors is probably multi-factorial. Doctors face barriers in accessing mental health care and work in stressful and often unsupportive environments with easy access to lethal drugs. More research is needed to explore trends in the rates of suicide among members of the medical profession, particularly women doctors who are up to four to six times more likely to commit suicide than women in the general population.

Recurrent thoughts about death or self-harm are a medical emergency in anyone. Many of us will experience depression and thoughts of self-harm during our professional lives. We must recognise the symptoms and seek urgent support and advice from our own trusted medical practitioner. We must also be more vigilant in supporting other colleagues who appear to be struggling. The easiest questions to ask are: 'Are you OK?', 'What can I do to support you through this difficult time?'.

It is extremely difficult to ask a colleague if they are considering harming themselves. For our patients we are comfortable with asking: 'Many people who feel this way feel like harming themselves; have you ever felt this way?'. When we suspect our colleagues and friends are at risk, it may be better to listen with our eyes and to ask: 'I need to know you are being looked after and you are safe.'

BEREAVEMENT

The truth is, though, that after any great loss there is no such thing as normal life. When life returns, 'normal' will feel different. Profound grief is not something we get over. In time, we get on, sometimes noticing with surprise how much life is still giving to us even while it has been taking so much away.

Stephanie Dowrick, contemporary psychotherapist

As doctors, like the rest of the population, we can experience intense emotional reactions after bereavement including crying, irritability, worry, anger, guilt, insomnia, loss of interest in usual activities, depression and anxiety. Grief is more likely to be severe if there is a history of mental illness, a lack of social support and an unexpected or violent death of a loved one, especially a spouse or a child.

We need to accept that everyone reacts differently to grief. While some people are unable to concentrate on normal activities, others will wish to continue working. Each person's reaction is normal and should not be judged as pathological just because it differs from the reactions of other people.

At a time of bereavement it is OK to allow ourselves to cry and to talk about our feelings. It is OK to expose ourselves to sad memories but it sometimes helps to try to do this in a graded way and also to focus on positive and happy memories.

It is important to seek supportive relationships with family members and close friends because prolonged grief may result in depression, which could require ongoing treatment with formal psychotherapy and antidepressant medication. We must avoid the temptation of self-prescribing benzodiazepines and should consult with our own doctor if we feel we need assistance.

It is only when we make time for deep reflection that we will work through grief and emerge stronger. As the novelist V.S. Naipaul, winner of the Nobel Prize for Literature in 2001, said:

Grief never leaves you but it mutates into a deepening awareness of the greater capacity for love, and an extraordinary awareness of the interconnectedness of life.

A LIFE-THREATENING ILLNESS

Many of us remember thinking we might have the symptoms of one of the many serious illnesses we learned about during our early years as medical students. Over the years we tend to develop a healthy level of denial of personal illness, which may be one of the reasons we are so reluctant to consult our own doctors.

But when doctors are actually diagnosed with a life-threatening illness, many of us experience those old feelings of heightened anxiety because we know too much about options, possibilities and risks. We are likely to gain access to our investigation results before our own doctor. Patient brochures only give us limited information and we tend to spend our time on searches of the international medical literature studying the options of treatment when it would probably be better to spend time seeking the support of friends and family.

Our medical friends tend to ask us about our 'stage' and prognosis and other details of our disorder, rather than offering support or an opportunity to express our feelings. Our colleagues fully understand the reality of our answers and may then find it difficult to continue the conversation.

Our non-medical friends may tell us just to think positively as they know many people with similar illnesses who have survived. This superficial theory reflects a lack of understanding and unwillingness of others to confront serious illness. Unfortunately doctor patients can recount many stories of their own patients who have not survived their illness.

Our interactions with the health system can be very different when we are the patient. Our late friend and colleague Professor Chris Silagy described his experience with lymphoma like this:

Being a doctor does not guarantee easy access to good advice and appropriate medical treatment. I have learned to respect the skill and compassion of the oncology nurses. On many occasions they have made the difference to how I feel. I have also learned that a similar caring and compassionate approach is essential and desperately needed among medical staff. I have been fortunate to have some outstanding clinicians involved in my care. But I have also had my share of arrogant, insensitive and clinically atrocious doctors (right through from interns to senior consultants). This experience has impressed on me the need for doctors to really listen to their patients. As my lymphoma has gone through remissions and relapses, I have usually been the first person to detect the new small nodes or lesions. At times I have had to almost plead with the medical staff to take notice of my symptoms. Ironically, at one point I was so determined to prove that I was right,

I designed a small study on myself to confirm the findings and then published them in The Lancet![1]

Being a doctor patient can also be an advantage. We know how to access evidence-based health information, navigate the health system assertively and seek the best specialist care promptly. We gain a new understanding of the fear and powerlessness experienced by our patients. We gain a new understanding of the value of good communication and simple questions like 'How are you feeling?' and 'How can I support you?'.

> *Facing a personal crisis is a life challenge for anyone, but personal pain can be a wonderful teacher. For doctors, it is associated with special challenges that require special care from close family, friends and other colleagues. It is essential to find a doctor or other health professional we trust and then to trust their judgment. It is never easy to allow others to see us when we are vulnerable and to ask for support. When we do, we open ourselves to experiencing the profound love and kindness of others. We may then ask ourselves why we waited for a personal crisis to happen before we did so.*

---

1   Professor Chris Silagy (2001), 'A view from the other side: A doctor's experience of lymphoma', <www.racgp.org.au/gphealth/doctorsexperience>.

CHAPTER 12

EIGHT PRINCIPLES FOR BEING A RESILIENT DOCTOR

To laugh often and much,
To win the respect of intelligent people
And the affection of children,
To earn the appreciation of honest critics,
And to endure the betrayal of false friends,
To appreciate beauty,
To find the best in others,
To leave the world a bit better,
Whether by a healthy child, a garden patch
Or a redeemed social condition,
To know even one life has breathed easier
Because you live,
This is to have succeeded.
Ralph Waldo Emerson (1803–1882), poet and philosopher

Medicine is a rewarding and endlessly challenging career. Hanging in there for the long haul requires the ability to transcend adversity. When we consider all the complex issues we juggle every day, sometimes it seems easier to try to ignore the frustration and just get on with the job. But chronic states of stress can catch up with us and if this happens patient care will suffer.

EIGHT PRINCIPLES FOR BEING A RESILIENT DOCTOR

Make home a sanctuary.

Value strong relationships.

Have an annual preventive health assessment.

Control stress, not people.

Recognise conflict as an opportunity.

Manage bullying and violence assertively.

Make our medical organisations work for us.

Create a legacy.

Most importantly we need to challenge our medical culture which tends to encourage us to wear our state of chronic stress like a badge of honour. For these reasons, all of us need to think about ways to maintain our own resilience in the long term and how we care for our colleagues.

In this book, we have advocated that looking after ourselves and building strong relationships is an essential component of providing competent medical care to our patients. In this final chapter, we discuss eight principles for being a resilient doctor.

MAKE HOME A SANCTUARY

In any demanding career, it is essential to have a quiet sanctuary away from work. It is sometimes difficult to nurture personal relationships when working long hours or when working in different locations. It is tempting to withdraw from contact with family and friends on the weekends if we have been interacting with hundreds of people during the week. While making time for solitude is important for self-renewal, withdrawing socially from people regularly is a sign of burnout, which can lead to mental health problems. Unfortunately doctors experience high levels of marital and sexual disharmony with partners, often due to the excessive demands of work.

We can proactively choose partnerships and friendships which energise us and provide mutual love and support. As doctors we often find ourselves adopting our carer role in our personal relationships as well as our professional lives. While this is inevitable, it is also important to seek out people who will help sustain us.

We need to be aware of the pitfalls of parenting and the challenges of balancing the responsibilities of a parent with a busy professional life. We need to choose the parenting style that protects our children and allows them to grow into healthy, autonomous adults.

By caring for our families and friends, we create a welcoming sanctuary at home—a place to relax and restore ourselves and our loved ones.

VALUE STRONG RELATIONSHIPS

Strong doctors have strong relationships. As doctors we face excessive demands on a daily basis. To get the job done, many of us try to manage each day by unsuccessfully attempting to complete endless 'tick lists' at the expense of our professional and personal relationships. We need to take time every day also to nurture healthy relationships with ourselves, our family and friends, our patients, our colleagues and our physical environment.

Anyone with the right training and experience can become an excellent medical technician. What sets excellent doctors apart are their strong, caring relationships with people.

HAVE AN ANNUAL PREVENTIVE HEALTH ASSESSMENT

As doctors, we each need our own doctor, someone whom we trust for our own medical care and advice. If we are going to prevent major health problems, we must attend our own doctor for regular evidence-based preventive health assessment to allow early identification and management of the symptoms and signs of any physical or mental illness. The early detection of serious illness saves lives and can prevent years of unnecessary suffering. As doctors, we deserve to have access to the same level of quality medical care that we provide to each of our own patients. Our families also deserve this standard of care. Organise for a check-up today with a trusted colleague.

CONTROL STRESS, NOT PEOPLE

As doctors, we tend to have reputations for being overcontrolling. Whether this is true or not, many of us tend to develop driven personalities as an adaptation to the demands of our work. This personality can be a positive in the workplace, but can be damaging in our personal lives.

We need to accept that other people can't be controlled and allow others to learn from the consequences of their actions. We need to learn to delegate and share care more effectively. Sometimes our patients, particularly those with special needs, benefit from a multidisciplinary team approach rather than the services of a single doctor working in isolation.

It is important to maintain feelings of control over our lives by managing the stresses we do have control over. Ignoring problems will not make them go away. Stress should not be worn like a 'badge of honour'. We can take time to address the background stresses in our lives and to transcend difficulties by:

- Understanding our driven personalities and learning to take a break from these traits
- Recognising and addressing signs and causes of chronic negative stress
- Leveraging time and delegating tasks
- Challenging our own negative thinking and beliefs
- Aiming for wellbeing, rather than absence of stress.

RECOGNISE CONFLICT AS AN OPPORTUNITY

This is not about seeking or avoiding conflict. It's about managing conflict maturely when it inevitably arises.

In order to deal effectively with conflict, we can recognise it as an opportunity to build stronger relationships with people. If we have ever had a calm debate with someone over an important issue that concludes in a negotiated solution, we will recognise that our relationship with that person has become stronger. If we have ever amicably agreed to disagree with someone over an issue, we will recognise that the ability to have an open debate, even without resolution, has strengthened our relationship with that person.

On the other hand, avoiding conflict, non-assertiveness, hyper-sensitivity to criticism, refusing to listen or angrily squashing another person's point of view can be destructive to relationships.

We can become as expert at managing challenging behaviours and strong personalities, conflict and anger as we are with managing other aspects of our professional work. We can learn how to deal with criticism constructively.

MANAGE BULLYING AND VIOLENCE ASSERTIVELY

Bullying and violence are not acceptable behaviours and must not be tolerated. As doctors, we must know our responsibilities as employers in addressing cases of bullying or violence in the workplace. We need to be aware of how our own behaviours are perceived and strive always to behave in an appropriate professional manner.

Medical practitioners must become skilled in ways of assertively managing patient-initiated violence and violent behaviour must always be reported to the police. Failure to do this often results in the violence being deflected onto another colleague or onto the wider community.

It is well known that people with mental illness suffer a great deal because of the stigma attached to their disorder and they are more likely to be the victims rather than the perpetrators of violence. People with mental illness are overrepresented in the criminal justice system and this is a major worldwide human rights issue. It is our responsibility to advocate for better access by our patients to optimal mental health care.

MAKE OUR MEDICAL ORGANISATIONS WORK FOR US

Our medical organisations are charged with the responsibility of advocating about many of the issues that affect our ability to deliver a high-quality service to our patients and our communities. These issues may range from areas of clinical interest, inequity in access to health care, clinical independence, training needs or the impact of the environment on health. By becoming involved in our membership organisations, even in a limited way, we can gain peer support, develop areas of special interest and learn how our organisations work and how our organisations can provide us with ongoing support and advice. Our medical organisations can also provide opportunities for leadership training to support our roles in advocating for our communities and our patients.

CREATE A LEGACY

We can be proud of our profession. Each of us has the potential to be a role model for future doctors and contribute our own lasting legacy through the examples we set in the way we live our lives and practise medicine.

It may be worth considering how each of us would like to be remembered at the end of our medical careers and act accordingly now. Each of us has a set of values and principles which determine how we behave as ethical medical practitioners. In creating our legacy we can also discover ways to transcend adversity that we encounter as part of our professional lives.

It helps to focus on big-picture issues that make a difference by:

- Finding meaning and purpose in our everyday work and rediscovering the joy of being a doctor.
- Identifying the qualities we admire in our role models, mentors and colleagues.
- Upholding our integrity in everything we do.
- Developing goals for all aspects of our lives including our spiritual life, our physical and mental health, our careers and our relationships with other people, especially those who love and support us.
- Personally supporting our medical and other colleagues.

Through our experience as doctors we learn how to deal effectively with the many great joys and the many challenges of medical life. In this book, we have shared some of the principles we have learned about protecting ourselves from harm and developing resilience. Most importantly, our patients and our colleagues have taught us about the true meaning of healing.

In writing about healing from an Aboriginal perspective, Professor Helen Milroy, a child and adolescent psychiatrist and Australia's first Indigenous doctor, provides an inspirational example for us all:

Healing is part of life and continues through death and into life again. It occurs throughout a person's life journey as well as across generations. It can be experienced in many forms such as mending a wound or recovery from an illness. Mostly however it is about renewal. Leaving behind those things that have wounded us and caused us pain. Moving forward in our journey with hope for the future, with renewed energy, strength and enthusiasm for life. Healing gives us back to ourselves. Not to hide or fight anymore. But to sit still, calm our minds, listen to the universe and allow our spirits to dance on the wind. It lets us enjoy the sunshine and be bathed by the golden glow of the moon as we drift into our dreamtime. Healing ultimately gives us back to our country. To stand again on our rightful place, eternal and generational. Healing is not just about recovering what has been lost or repairing what has been broken. It is about embracing our life force to create a new and vibrant fabric that keeps us grounded and connected, wraps us in warmth and love and gives us the joy of seeing what we have created. Healing keeps us strong and gentle at the same time. It gives us balance and harmony, a place of triumph and sanctuary for evermore.

While 'first do no harm' has long referred to protecting our patients, in the 21st century its meaning needs to be expanded to also include protecting our families, our colleagues, our environment and ourselves.

If we are going to be effective medical practitioners providing care to each of our patients and contributing to healthier and stronger communities, we must not only avoid inadvertently harming ourselves, but be proactive in building our resilience. We must learn about the true meaning of healing.

CHECKLISTS FOR MENTAL HEALTH PROBLEMS

Reprinted with permission from *beyondblue*: the national depression initiative (Australia). <www.beyondblue.org.au>

DEPRESSION

For more than TWO WEEKS have you:

☐ Felt sad, down or miserable most of the time?

☐ Lost interest or pleasure in most of your usual activities?

If you answered 'YES' to any of these questions, complete the symptom checklist below. If you did not answer 'YES' to either of these questions, it is unlikely that you have a depressive illness.

☐ Lost or gained a lot of weight OR had a decrease or increase in appetite?

☐ Sleep disturbance?

☐ Felt slowed down, restless or excessively busy?

☐ Felt tired or had no energy?

☐ Felt worthless, excessively guilty or felt guilty about things without a good reason?

☐ Had poor concentration OR had difficulties thinking OR were very indecisive?

☐ Had recurrent thoughts of death?

Add up the number of ticks in your total score. What does your score mean? (Assuming you answered 'YES' to question 1 and/or question 2)

4 or less: You are unlikely to be experiencing a depressive illness.

5 or more: It is likely that you may be experiencing a depressive illness.

GENERALISED ANXIETY DISORDER

☐ For SIX MONTHS or more on more days than not, have you felt very worried

☐ found it hard to stop worrying

☐ found that your anxiety made it difficult for you to do everyday activities (e.g. work, study, seeing friends and family)?

If you answered 'YES' to ALL of these questions have you also experienced THREE or more of the following:

☐ felt restless or on edge

☐ felt easily tired

☐ had difficulty concentrating

☐ felt irritable

☐ had muscle pain (e.g. sore jaw or back)

☐ had trouble sleeping (e.g. difficulty falling or staying asleep or restless sleep)?

If you answered 'YES' it is important to see your own doctor:

PANIC DISORDER

Within a 10-MINUTE PERIOD have you felt FOUR OR MORE of the following:

☐ shaky

☐ increased heart rate

☐ short of breath

☐ choked

☐ nausea or pain in the stomach

☐ dizzy, lightheaded or faint

☐ numb or tingly

☐ derealisation (feelings of unreality) or depersonalisation
   (feeling detached from yourself or your surroundings)

☐ hot or cold flushes

☐ scared of going crazy

☐ scared of dying?

If you answered 'YES' to FOUR OR MORE of these questions, have you also: felt scared, for ONE MONTH OR MORE, of experiencing these feelings again?

If you answered 'YES' it is important to see your own doctor.

POST-TRAUMATIC STRESS DISORDER

Have you:

☐ experienced or seen something that involved death, injury, torture or abuse and felt very scared or helpless

☐ had upsetting memories or dreams of the event for at least ONE month

☐ found it hard to go about your daily life (e.g. made it difficult for you to work/study or get along with family and friends)?

If you answered 'YES' to ALL of these questions, have you also experienced at least THREE of the following:

☐ avoided activities that remind you of the event

☐ had trouble remembering parts of the event

☐ felt less interested in doing things you used to enjoy

☐ had trouble feeling intensely positive emotions (e.g. love or excitement)

☐ thought less about the future (e.g. about career or family goals)?

☐ AND have you experienced at least TWO of the following:

☐ had difficulties sleeping (e.g. had bad dreams, or found it hard to fall or stay asleep)

☐ felt easily angry or irritated

☐ had trouble concentrating

☐ felt on guard

☐ been easily startled?

If you answered 'YES', it is important to see your own doctor.

OBSESSIVE COMPULSIVE DISORDER

Have you:

☐ had repetitive thoughts or concerns that are not simply about real life problems (e.g. thoughts that you or people close to you will be harmed)

☐ done the same activity repeatedly and in a very ordered, precise and similar way each time e.g.: constantly washing your hands or clothes, showering or brushing your teeth, constantly cleaning, tidying or rearranging in a particular way things at home, at work or in the car, constantly checking that doors and windows are locked and/or appliances are turned off

☐ felt relieved in the short term by doing these things, but soon felt the need to repeat them?

☐ recognised that these feelings, thoughts and behaviours were unreasonable?

☐ found that these thoughts or behaviours take up more than 1 hour a day and/or interfered with your normal routine (e.g. working, studying or seeing friends and family)?

If you answered 'YES' it is important to see your own doctor.

PHOBIA

Have you felt very nervous when faced with a specific object or situation e.g.:

☐ flying on an airplane

☐ going near an animal

☐ receiving an injection

☐ going to a social event?

Have you avoided a situation that might cause you to face the phobia e.g.:

☐ needed to change work patterns

☐ not attending social events

☐ not getting health check-ups

☐ found it hard to go about your daily life (e.g. working, studying or seeing friends and family) because you are trying to avoid such situations?

If you answered 'YES' it is important to see your own doctor.

REFERENCES

(1) American Psychiatric Association (1994), *Diagnostic and Statistical Manual of Mental Disorders*, 4th edn (DSM-IV), Washington DC: APA; and (2) *International Classification of Diseases and Related Health Problems*, 10th revision, Geneva, World Health Organization, 1992–1994.

RECOMMENDED READING

Clarke, J. (2005), *Monster at Work*, Sydney: Random House.

Frankl, V. (1984), *Man's Search for Meaning*, New York: Washington Square Press.

Kay, M., Mitchell, G., Clavarino, A., Danst, J., *Doctors as patients: a systematic review of doctors' health access and the barriers they experience*, British Journal of General Practice, July 2008.

McGrath, H. and Edwards, H. (2000), *Difficult Personalities*, Marrickville, NSW: Choice Books.

Piterman, L., Hassed, C. and Piterman, H. (2007), *GP Self Care: Chapter in General Practice Psychiatry*, edited by Grant Blashki, Fiona Judd and Leon Piterman, Sydney: McGraw-Hill Australia, pp15–31.

Rowe, L. and Kidd, M. (2007), *Save your life and the lives of those you love: Your GP's 6 step guide to staying healthy longer*, Sydney: Allen & Unwin.

Royal Australian College of General Practitioners (2003), *The Conspiracy of Silence*, Melbourne: RACGP.

Royal Australian College of General Practitioners (2005), *Keeping the Doctor Alive*, Melbourne: RACGP.

Doctors' Health and Lifestyle, *Medical Journal of Australia*, (2004) 181 (7) www.mja.com.au/public/issues/181_07_041004/contents_041004.html

WHO-WONCA report (2008) *Integrating mental health into primary care—A global perspective*, WHO Press, World Health Organization, Geneva, Switzerland.

INDEX